A Light in the Tower

RETHINKING CAREERS, RETHINKING ACADEMIA
Joseph Fruscione and Erin Bartram, *Series Editors*

A Light in the Tower

A New Reckoning with Mental Health in Higher Education

KATIE ROSE GUEST PRYAL

University Press of Kansas

Published by the University Press of Kansas (Lawrence, Kansas 66045), which was organized by the Kansas Board of Regents and is operated and funded by Emporia State University, Fort Hays State University, Kansas State University, Pittsburg State University, the University of Kansas, and Wichita State University.

Library of Congress Cataloging-in-Publication Data

Names: Pryal, Katie Rose Guest, author.
Title: A light in the tower : a new reckoning with mental health in higher education / Katie Rose Guest Pryal.
Description: Lawrence, Kansas : University Press of Kansas, [2024] | Series: Rethinking careers, rethinking academia | Includes bibliographical references.
Identifiers: LCCN 2023029009 (print) | LCCN 2023029010 (ebook)
ISBN 9780700636358 (cloth)
ISBN 9780700636334 (paperback)
ISBN 9780700636341 (ebook)
Subjects: LCSH: College teachers—Mental health—United States. | College students—Mental health—United States. | Universities and colleges—Employees—Mental health—United States. | People with mental disabilities—Education (Higher)—United States. | Education, Higher—United States—Psychological aspects.
Classification: LCC LB2333.2 .P794 2024 (print) | LCC LB2333.2 (ebook) | DDC 378.1/2—dc23/eng/20231115
LC record available at https://lccn.loc.gov/2023029009.
LC ebook record available at https://lccn.loc.gov/2023029010.

British Library Cataloguing-in-Publication Data is available.

Printed in the United States of America

The paper used in this publication is acid free and meets the minimum requirements of the American National Standard for Permanence of Paper for Printed Library Materials Z39.48-1992.

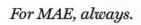

For MAE, always.

Content Warning

Some people, like me, need content warnings to allow us to fully engage with and appreciate our world, including books.

This book contains stories about self-harm, including death by suicide, descriptions of first-person experiences with mental health struggles, including depression and anxiety, stories of campus violence, and descriptions of bodily harm.

Contents

Preface

This is not a pandemic book.

The campus mental health crisis has been an ongoing problem for decades. We can, however, learn a lot by examining how the pandemic shined a spotlight on campus mental health. During the pandemic, mental health in higher education communities rapidly deteriorated. Even now, years since the start of the pandemic, our communities have not recovered. But I want to ask, *recovered from what?* From the pandemic? Or from decades of neglect by higher education institutions?

The answer is the second.

Yes, the pandemic wrought immense stressors on higher education communities. Classes suddenly shifted to online teaching and learning, then shifted back to campus while COVID still loomed large. Faculty faced intense labor conditions, particularly vulnerable faculty, including those who are marginalized or have little job security. Vulnerable faculty in particular had to do immense caretaking of students. Students faced new, intense stress at a time in their lives when they were leaving behind their support systems, and they continued to face stress as many professors expected them to act as though their entire worlds had not been upended.

Yet before COVID, faculty already faced intense labor conditions with the decades-long shift of higher education to a market-driven model that demands overwhelming production by faculty, driving them to overwork, to burnout, and to anxiety, depression, and worse.[1] Vulnerable faculty have always faced the immense burden of student carework that goes far beyond their job descriptions.[2] And students have always faced mental health strain when they leave for college, upending their lives and struggling to navigate not only frequently unreasonable educational expectations, but life expectations as well.

This strain is even greater for students with mental disabilities (such as autism, ADHD, and anxiety), who must navigate a new learning environment that is hostile to those very disabilities. This hostility derives from stigma, and the stigma against mental disabilities in academia is particularly harsh. It also has a ripple effect that poisons the entire higher education community.

The Stigma Against Mental Disability in Higher Education

I define stigma against mentally disabled people as a process that creates negative stereotyping and isolation, typically based on the irrational fear of undesirable behavior such as irresponsibility, instability, or violence. Stigma also works internally on disabled people, creating feelings of isolation and shame.

Stigma causes higher education communities to systematically mistreat students and faculty with mental disabilities. For example, it causes community members to feel suspicious that students with ADHD are faking their diagnoses in order to cheat. It causes faculty and other community members to feel an irrational fear of students and colleagues with bipolar disorder. It causes universities to force students with depression or other mental health struggles to withdraw from college altogether because of lack of support.[3]

Mental disability remains stigmatized despite its prevalence in higher education. Long before the pandemic, higher education had high rates of mental disability. For example, in a 2018 study, 39 percent of faculty and staff and 42 percent of undergraduates screened positive for anxiety.[4] By comparison, the National Institute for Mental Health reports that 19 percent of US adults have anxiety.[5]

Stigma against mental disabilities causes students and faculty who develop these struggles after entering academia—as these numbers show, there are many—to avoid treatment because they do not want to be stigmatized too. Therefore, stigma makes it difficult, sometimes impossible, for academic communities to effectively address mental health issues.

Why does mental disability remain so firmly stigmatized within the ivory tower? As I wrote many years ago, "Academia isn't an easy place to be if your brain isn't quite right."[6] I have bipolar disorder, anxiety disorder, and autism spectrum disorder, which means I am a mentally disabled person in a workplace that makes clear, in ways large and small, that I do not belong. Why? I explained, "We are, in academia, still devoted to the mythos of the good human speaking well, the professor as a bastion of reason, the *cogito ergo sum*."[7] Based on the logic of academia, if my brain is wrong, then *everything* about me is wrong. As disability studies scholar Margaret Price points out, students and faculty with mental disabilities "are largely excluded from academic discourse."[8] That is, they are not fully fledged members of the academic community; they are pushed to the margins.

If you are mentally disabled in higher education, evidence shows that you cannot expect to be listened to or believed. In an essay on how our society—including the medical profession and higher education—does not let autistic people speak for themselves, disability studies scholar M. Remi Yergeau, who is autistic and uses the pronouns they/them, tells the story of how, during their second week as a professor, they were involuntarily committed to a psychiatric facility. They were strapped to a gurney and wheeled out of an academic building on campus, a terrifying and humiliating experience. They tried to reason with their colleagues, the EMTs, and other people around them, telling everyone that they did not need inpatient psychiatric care, but no one listened to them. Instead, others at the scene attributed Yergeau's words to their disabilities. Yergeau describes the responses: "'That's your depression talking,' they explained. 'That's your autism talking. That's your anxiety talking. Really, it's anything but you talking.'"[9] As Yergeau's story shows, mentally disabled faculty are always at risk of losing their agency, their control over their decision-making, their control over their lives—over their *everything*. Yergeau explains the problem succinctly: "I am the ultimate unreliable narrator." Given the risks to our safety, it is no wonder that so many of us keep our mental disabilities hidden, if we are privileged enough to have disabilities that allow us to do so.

In short, our society, and particularly higher education, sees any brain that deviates from a normal brain as wrong, or as broken. The great joke of it all is that there is no normal brain. But even though the normal brain is a social construct, in the world we live in, there are normates—nondisabled people—and then there is us.

COVID has brought the stigma against mental disability into focus because so many more people are now struggling with their mental health; we have reached a critical mass that institutions can no longer ignore. Writing on "collective trauma" events such as COVID, faculty development professional and neurodiversity expert Karen Ray Costa, who has ADHD, points out, "On one hand, [collective trauma events] are horrifying and destructive. But on the other, they often prompt 'a crisis of meaning' that leads groups and individuals to imagine new, possible worlds."[10] Imagine higher education without stigma against mental disabilities. In this new higher education system, disability accommodations do not require anything more than a person asking for them, instead of heaps of invasive and expensive paperwork required by a culture eternally suspicious of disabled people. Imagine a higher education system where every course and meeting is accessible. Imagine a student or colleague in a mental health crisis being unafraid to ask for help and having help readily accessible. These are possible outcomes if administrators are courageous enough to take the required steps. As Costa writes, why should we want to return to normal? After all, "the old normal sucked for a lot of people . . . why would we want more of the same?"[11] We don't. We want a better world.

Labor and Mental Disability

Labor adds another complex layer to mental disability and higher education. With the rise of the market-driven university came the rise of contingent labor—contract faculty who are paid little and have little job security. This shift began decades ago but has now reached the point where nearly 75 percent of all undergraduate courses are taught by contingent faculty.[12]

Because so many faculty are not "professors" in the arcane job-title terminology of academia, I have deliberately opted against using such terminology in this book. It only serves to stratify, and therefore justify the mistreatment and overwork of those at the bottom of those stratifications.[13] Therefore, when I use the term "faculty," I am referring to all higher education workers who are responsible for the education of students, be they librarians, academic support professionals, student advisers, classroom teachers on or off the tenure track, and more. Furthermore, I refer to all classroom teachers as "professors" because their job duties are to teach, and that is what professors do.

In higher education circles, contingent faculty are referred to by a variety of terms: non-tenure-track faculty, adjuncts, precarious faculty, contract faculty, and more. For continuity's sake, when necessary, I will refer to these faculty as "contingent faculty."

I've spent my entire career as a contingent faculty member, off the tenure track, on tenuous renewable contracts, with a job that was always insecure. My fellow contingent faculty and I used to joke that we were "fake professors." We were not, of course, but that is how the administration and our tenured colleagues frequently made us feel. The point is, I had insecure employment. But contingent labor frequently intersects with mental disability to make the employment status of mentally disabled academics even more insecure.[14]

Why I Wrote This Book

I wrote this book to end stigma against mentally disabled people in higher education—and everywhere.

If higher education institutions want to effectively address the mental health crisis on campus, it must end the stigma against mental disabilities and create an environment that is inclusive of mentally disabled people.

The typical definition of inclusion refers to giving equal access to opportunities to people who would otherwise be excluded. Based on this definition, you could think that inclusion means merely opening the door—"Here, you have access now." But that mentality puts the burden on the excluded group to enter a place that has previously been hostile. Therefore, my definition is this: inclusion of mentally disabled people means removing any burdens to join a community that has previously stigmatized them by taking active steps to welcome them.

I am trained as a lawyer (JD) and a rhetorician (PhD), which means I am an expert in public discourse and how it influences policy. I am also an expert in disability studies, in particular the study of mental disabilities. I am mentally disabled: I have bipolar disorder and anxiety disorder, and I am autistic. My specific training, skills, and identity have helped me write a book that is grounded in praxis: it binds the testimony of my experience as a mentally disabled person with research in order to support a call for policy change.

What I have found while writing this book are three cascading facts:

(1) Mental disability is stigmatized in higher education.

(2) This stigma against mental disabilities prevents higher education from reckoning with its mental health crisis because it pushes mental health struggles to the shadows.

(3) The inclusion of mentally disabled faculty and students, which will break the stigma against mental disability, is the only solution to the campus mental health crisis.

This book does its work through various lenses: my experience as a mentally disabled person and as a professor; interviews with professors, students, and mentally disabled people; and scholarly and popular research.

My hope is that this book will push higher education closer to destigmatizing mental disability and toward treating mentally disabled people with respect, kindness, and collegiality. If higher education communities can set aside their fears surrounding mental disability, they can advocate rather than isolate. They can finally bring light to the shadowed corners of the ivory tower.

Book Overview

This book is divided into two parts. The first gives an overview of the mental health crisis facing higher education. The second focuses on how to teach while reckoning with mental disability.

Following this preface is an introduction, "How to Talk about Mental Disability." It introduces the book by way of a living glossary of terms related to mental disability (including "mental disability" itself). Its driving premise is this: how we talk about mental disability affects how we treat mentally disabled people.

Part I, "The Mental Health Crisis in Higher Education," tackles the large-scale mental health challenges that faculty and students face. I use the mental health struggles brought to light during the pandemic only to highlight the struggles that were already there, hiding in the shadows. These struggles include academic burnout, the prevalence of anxiety disorders in higher education, and academia's toxic overwork problem. These chapters validate the difficulties faced by mentally disabled people. They also reach out to readers who are facing new mental health struggles and are unsure of how to seek help. They speak to readers who wish to be allies and those with influence to make positive institutional changes to inclusion and to break down stigma.

Part II, "Teaching with Mental Health in Mind," addresses student depression and suicide, which have been ignored far too long and which the pandemic has helped bring to light (finally). It takes on the mental health stigma students face and what faculty can do about it. It talks about what I have dubbed "rigor angst," the irrational fear that a curriculum will not be difficult enough to meet academic standards. Rigor angst has come to the fore during the pandemic—although it has been around for as long as there have been students. It arises from a deep well of mistrust toward students, particularly students struggling with their mental health. This part gives advice for teaching accessibly and inclusively, including strategies for teaching mentally disabled students, understanding procrastination, creating student mental health communities, and using attendance as a teaching tool rather than a punishment. Part II shows how teaching accessibly and inclusively is better for disabled students, and all students.

Introduction

How to Talk about Mental Disability

As I introduce this book on mental health and disability, I want to tell you where I'm coming from. I am not a therapist or a doctor. I don't conduct research on human subjects. No, I am a law professor with a doctorate in rhetoric who specializes in disability studies. Being a rhetorician and law professor means that I am an expert in how public discourse affects public policy. And *that* means that I am an expert in how what we say every day becomes the laws that govern our society.

(It also means I spend a lot of time explaining what I do to people.)

I also have bipolar disorder and anxiety disorder, and I am autistic. So when I talk about what it means to have a mental disability, or to be stigmatized for it, I am speaking from experience.

My research lab is in the public sphere, where pundits, lobbyists, and politicians address spree killings on television with talk about "good guys with guns"—and with those words they mean the opposite of people like me, because people like me "need to be committed, is what they need to be."[1] My lab is also quiet corners of the faculty lounge, when I am with colleagues and one says, "You know how bipolar the dean is!" and everyone laughs because "bipolar" is a joke, not a diagnosis, and if you can't take a joke you're a downer. And although the words may be a joke, they have a material effect on me and every other mentally disabled person who hears them. They also have a material effect on normates who hear them. For disabled people, these words give us no reason to trust that we will be treated as fully human. For normates, these words give tacit permission to treat disabled people as subhuman. In short, these words, these *jokes*, enforce the stigma against mental disabilities that rots the core of our communities.

What I've learned over the past twenty years of doing this work is that how we—in the most public of places or the most private—*talk* about mental disability affects how we—our society at large or our smallest communities—*treat* mentally disabled people.

You might not have given much thought to the language of mental disability, mental illness, mental health, neurodiversity, psychiatry, and so on. Our society has come a long way from the R-word, but there is still a big gap between avoiding slurs and speaking thoughtfully. As disability activist and author Emily Landau explains, "Language is one of the most important signals that we have to demonstrate our acceptance or rejection of a person's identity."[2] Thus, how we talk about mentally disabled people can justify exclusion and even abuse, or it can create inclusion and acceptance.

So when we talk about disability, we must presume, always, that we are talking with disabled people even if we don't realize it. We must presume, also, that our language changes how every person, normate and disabled alike, thinks about disabled people. At its best, language can be liberatory. In the case of mentally disabled people, who have been and continue to be excluded, confined, and incarcerated simply because of our disabilities, I use "liberatory" not only metaphorically but also quite literally.

There are many terms having to do with mental disability that might seem to refer to the same things, for example, "mental health," "mental illness," "neurodivergence," "psychiatric disability," and "mental disability." Although some of these terms overlap, they do not mean the same thing, and they can be confusing. If you are new to this vocabulary, you might be uncomfortable talking about mental disability because you are afraid of making a mistake.

I can think of no better way to introduce a book about mental health and disability than with a tool to help talk about mental health and disability. Here, I hope to allay confusion and help create a language of inclusion. In doing so, I aim to use the words preferred by most disabled writers and activists. But the fact is, language constantly evolves. This introduction, then, is fixed in the time that I have written it. In ten years, some of my words may be relics. Creating a language of inclusion is an ongoing process as we, disabled people, continuously discover who we are and who we want to be. Furthermore, mentally disabled people are not a monolithic group, so our perspectives on language differ.

Please take this introduction for what it is: a starting point for everyone to feel more comfortable talking about mental disability.

Mental Illness

The term "mental illness" seems fairly straightforward since it is a phrase in the common parlance. The American Psychiatric Association (APA) defines mental illnesses as "health conditions involving changes in emotion, thinking or behavior (or a combination of these). Mental illnesses are associated with distress and/or difficulty functioning in social, work or family activities."[3] When I am talking about myself, I use this term to refer to my diagnoses of bipolar disorder and generalized anxiety disorder. The APA emphasizes, "Mental illness is treatable." The ability to treat mental illness is what distinguishes it from other types of mental disabilities, such as developmental disorders, as I discuss later. (This distinction is debatable, as I also discuss later.)

The APA demarcates between mental illness and "serious" mental illness. They note that just over 4 percent of US adults have a "serious" mental illness in a given year. Serious mental illness, according to the APA, is a "mental, behavioral or emotional disorder (excluding developmental and substance use disorders) resulting in serious functional impairment, which substantially interferes with or limits one or more major life activities." What counts as a "serious" mental illness for the APA? They list "major depressive disorder, schizophrenia and bipolar disorder." Thus, with my diagnosis of bipolar disorder, I am in that 4 percent.

Mental illness is often contrasted with the term "mental health." The contrast is right there in the words themselves: if a person is mentally ill, the person ought to seek to be mentally healthy. But the idea of mental illness being faulty and mental health being the ultimate goal is fraught with problems.

Mental Health

The term "mental health" can cause insidious harm because it sanitizes the discussion of mental disability. We hear about mental health constantly (it is even in the title of this book) because it is a term that people feel more comfortable talking about. After all, mental health is something we all want and can support, right? Mental illness, on the other hand, is scary.

But there are problems with the term "mental health"—and with its companion "mental illness." First and foremost, they are terms of the medical establishment, not of disabled people ourselves. As disability scholar and advocate Margaret Price notes: "Mental health is the term of choice for the medical community as well as insurance companies and social support services."[4] Price explains that "mental health" creates a "well/unwell paradigm" that, in turn, creates an "implication that a mad person needs to be 'cured' by some means." (Note that Price is using the term *mad* in a nonderogatory fashion.) What is the problem with having "cure" as a goal? As Price explains, one problem is insurance coverage. Because "insurance operates on a 'cure' basis," companies frequently end coverage when the patient is deemed "well" enough, which may not correlate at all with the person's actual needs. The expectation of wellness bleeds over into our cultural expectations as well. Our society expects a depressed person to someday get better. For anxiety to go away. For mental illness to become mental wellness.

But some of us will never be cured because our disabilities are, by their nature, lifelong. For example, my bipolar disorder can be managed (and in that I am fortunate), but it will never go away. For many people, a cure is not in the cards, no matter how badly insurance companies wish it were so. Author and psychologist Andrew Solomon describes interactions with the public in which audiences are shocked that he continues to take medication for his chronic depression:

> I am often asked in social situations to describe my own experiences, and I usually end by saying that I am on medication. "Still?" people ask. "But you seem fine!" To which I invariably reply that I seem fine because I am fine, and that I am fine in part because of medication. . . . When I say that I will be on medication indefinitely, people who have dealt calmly and sympathetically with the news of suicide attempts, catatonia, missed years of work, significant loss of body weight, and so on stare at me with alarm. . . . "Surely now you are strong enough to be able to phase out some of these drugs!"[5]

Solomon's anecdote demonstrates our social norm of mental wellness, which does not accurately reflect the reality of living with mental

disability. In Solomon's case, the social norm of wellness equals no longer taking antidepressants because if you need antidepressants, you are
not "cured."

For all of these reasons, "mental health," as a term, can be a bogeyman for those of us with mental disabilities. It implies that we should
seek cures, even when cures do not exist. It implies that we are weak
(unable to "phase out some of these drugs") or broken because we have a
chronic illness and are therefore not "healthy." The term "mental health,"
then, should be used carefully. Recognize that mental wellness is not a
morally superior state of being. Rather, use the term "mental health"
to describe an element of bodily health that we can examine, without
judgment or stigma.

Developmental Disorders and Disabilities

According to The Centers for Disease Control and Prevention (CDC),
"Developmental disabilities are a group of conditions due to an impairment in physical, learning, language, or behavior areas. These conditions begin during the developmental period, may impact day-to-day
functioning, and usually last throughout a person's lifetime."[6] Developmental disabilities include autism spectrum disorder (ASD), attention
deficit and hyperactivity disorder (ADHD), and more.

Generally, medical professionals do not consider a developmental
disability a mental illness. Take, for example, autism. According to the
Mental Health Foundation (UK), "Autism is a developmental disability
that affects how people communicate and experience the world around
them. It isn't a mental health problem." The CDC defines autism as "a
developmental disability that can cause significant social, communication and behavioral challenges."[7]

The APA, CDC, and other medical organizations tend to draw a clear
demarcation between developmental disorders and mental illness. For
example, the Thompson Policy Institute on Disability provides this
distinction between developmental disabilities and mental illnesses:
"While intellectual and developmental disabilities (IDD's) [such as au-
tism] can slow cognitive ability among other processes, mental illnesses
alter cognitive perception without diminishing cognitive ability."[8] This
distinction is one you will find in many places: developmental disabilities slow cognitive ability; mental illnesses alter cognitive perception.

But in my work and my life, I have found that trying to draw a line between "mental illness" and a "developmental disorder" can be difficult. Take cognition, for example. When I am depressed, my cognitive abilities are essentially defunct. For example, in Chapter 8, "Writing Depression," I describe how my cognition is shut down by depression, a common occurrence for those who experience it. Psychiatric research has shown that depression can cause cognitive impairments, "which include deficits in various domains: attention, executive functions, memory and processing speed."[9] Similarly, when I am deeply anxious, I am unable to process information or make good decisions. In short, mental illness deeply affects my cognitive processes.

On the other hand, autism is a developmental disorder that supposedly affects my cognition, but I rarely notice it day to day. Take, for example, "working memory," which is "the retention of a small amount of information in a readily accessible form. It facilitates planning, comprehension, reasoning, and problem-solving."[10] Many autistics, including me, have weaker working memory when compared to our other cognitive traits.[11] (I do not mind calling this difference a "weakness"—because it is. All humans have them.) Because I have lived with this weakness my whole life, I have created workarounds to the point where it is rarely a cognitive weakness at all. If you asked me which of my mental disabilities affected my *cognition* the most, I would point to depression and anxiety before autism.

Thus, although the terms "mental illness" and "developmental disorder" are the preferred terms of the medical community, the demarcation between them frequently does not describe the lived experiences of mentally disabled people.

Neurodiversity

Neurodiversity refers to the range of differences in brain function and behavior that are part of the normal variation in the human population. As the Cleveland Clinic explains, "Neurodivergent is a nonmedical term that describes people whose brains develop or work differently for some reason. This means the person has different strengths and struggles from people whose brains develop or work more typically."[12] Importantly, they note, the umbrella of neurodivergence covers those who have not been diagnosed by traditional means: "While some people who are neurodivergent have medical conditions, it also happens to people where a medical condition or diagnosis hasn't been identified." In its best form, to me, neurodiversity is generous; for example, it includes those who have been self-diagnosed because a "real" diagnosis is too costly or otherwise unattainable.

The term "neurodiversity" is a portmanteau coined by Australian sociologist Judy Singer in 1998 with regard to autism: "For me, a key significance of the 'autism spectrum' lies in its call for and anticipation of a politics of neurological diversity, or neurodiversity."[13]Although Singer used the term in the context of autism spectrum disorder, in practice, it has had far-reaching effects for not only the autism rights movement but all neurodivergent people. You will sometimes see the term shortened to "ND."

Deriving from neurodiversity are the adjective "neurodivergent" and the noun "neurodivergence." Note that a person cannot be "neurodiverse" (or any other kind of "diverse"). Only a group of people can be so. When speaking about a person, use the word "neurodivergent." However, in common parlance today, you will see speakers and writers refer to an individual as "neurodiverse."

In a related fashion, you will see the word "neurotypical" (shortened to "NT"). Neurotypical refers to neurological development or behavior that is "normal" by societal standards. "Neurotypical" and "NT" are frequently used alongside "neurodivergent" and "ND" to refer to those who are neurodivergent and those who are not. These are safe, respectful terms.

You will also encounter the term "neuroatypical," which is the linguistic opposite of "neurotypical." Because this word is created in opposition to what is normal, it has negative connotations: "atypical" connotes abnormal, and abnormal connotes something *wrong*. "Neuroatypical" is, however, a term used in medical literature, so you will see it there.[14] But when speaking, use "neurodivergent" instead.

Over the years, I have frequently used "neurodivergent" as the umbrella term to refer to my own mental disabilities, because my disabilities span mental illness (bipolar disorder, anxiety disorder) and developmental disorder (autism). I am, indeed, neurodivergent. Although the word fits, it leaves out an important element, one I want to center in my identity and my work: disability. For that reason, in this book, I use the nearly synonymous term "mental disability," which I discuss next.

Psychiatric Disability and Mental Disability

"Psychiatric disability," although on its face a near-synonym for mental illness, provides a way to articulate mental illness as a disabled identity and not just as a medical problem to be treated. Before I was diagnosed with autism, a developmental disorder, in my forties, I only had diagnoses of mental illnesses: bipolar disorder and anxiety disorder. Thus, I referred to myself as psychiatrically disabled. The term "psychiatric disability," for me, and for many, creates a connection to the disabled community, a (usually) supportive community of people who care about each other and seek to make the world more accessible for all disabled people.

Not insignificantly, the term also brings legal and political power. Thus, if you have a serious mental illness (and some "nonserious" ones as well), you have the right to be recognized as disabled under the law and to receive certain protections and benefits.

But as I write about my disabilities now, the term "psychiatrically disabled" no longer fits. I now need a second term to refer to autism— because autism is not a psychiatric disability (a mental illness) but a developmental disorder. I have spent a long time searching for a term that encompasses both.

To bring together "neurodivergence," "mental illness," and "psychiatric disability," I now use a term Margaret Price introduced to me in her work: "mental disability."[15] Price writes, "This term [mental disability] can include not only madness, but also cognitive and intellectual dis/abilities of various kinds. I would add that it might also include 'physical' illnesses accompanied by mental effects (for example, the 'brain fog' that attends many autoimmune diseases, chronic pain, and chronic fatigue)." For me, "mental disability" encompasses the psychiatric, the developmental, and all other aspects of disability that have to do with the mind.

Framing mental illness as a disability provides a way to push back against "mental health" and "wellness" narratives. A disabled identity allows a person, if they wish, to reject the notion of a cure as a golden ring. They can, for example, more easily accept that they need antidepressants to live a good life, even if it means they are disabled forever, forever unhealed in the eyes of a wellness-centered society. As Ashe Grey, disability advocate and disability studies scholar, writes in her popular 2016 essay "Bad Crip," a "bad crip . . . doesn't think they need to be healed at all."[16]

To me, "mental disability" is a generous term. You will see it frequently in this book.

Normate, Neurotypical, Abled, and Ableism

There are various terms that refer to nondisabled people, psychiatrically or otherwise. The term I prefer is "normate," which can be an adjective or a noun. Thus, a person can be a "normate" (noun) or be "normate" (adjective). The term "normate" was coined by disability scholar Rosemarie Garland-Thomson in the 1990s. As she explains, normate is "the constructed identity of those who, by way of the bodily configurations and cultural capital they assume, can step into a position of authority and wield the power it grants them."[17] She coined the word "to defamiliarize the privileged designation of 'ablebodied,' shifting it out of the body and into the realm of social and political relations."[18] In other words, the term is intended to point out that being normate is about social norms and power. After all, as I've mentioned more than once in this chapter, what is "normal" is fluid.

The word "abled" is a synonym for "normate" and can also be an adjective or a noun. "Neurotypical" refers to people who are not neurodivergent. It is often shortened to "NT." None of these three terms is derogatory of people who are not disabled, although when disabled people are hurt or angry about mistreatment because of their disabilities, they sometimes discuss ableds or normates in angry tones. But in the end, the terms are used to identify; the terms themselves are not insults. I make this point because some normates take these terms to be insulting, as any group with political, institutional, or social power takes offense at merely being identified.

When disabled people talk about their mistreatment because of their disabilities, they are talking about ableism. Simply put, ableism is discrimination against disabled people in favor of abled people. Lydia X. Z. Brown provides a more comprehensive definition: "Ableism is systematic, institutional devaluing of bodies and minds deemed deviant, abnormal, defective, subhuman, less than."[19] In higher education, as Margaret Price explains, "ableism contributes to the construction of a rigid, elitist, hierarchical, and inhumane academic system."[20]

Stigma

Mental disabilities, in our society, are highly stigmatized. Stigma, in its most basic definition, means shame, or a mark of disgrace. I define stigma against mentally disabled people as a process that creates negative stereotyping and isolation, typically based on the irrational fear of undesirable behavior such as irresponsibility, instability, or violence. Stigma also works internally on disabled people themselves, creating feelings of isolation and shame.

Psychiatrist Bruce G. Link and sociologist Jo C. Phelan, in their foundational work on stigma and mental disabilities, describe it as a four-part process: dominant power structures (1) "distinguish and label" human differences (e.g., mental disabilities); (2) use cultural beliefs to mark those labeled differences as "undesirable"; (3) isolate the people with the undesirable characteristics; and (4) cause the isolated people to experience "disapproval, rejection, exclusion, and discrimination," thereby losing "access to social, economic, and political power."[21] Stigma and ableism work together, as stigma justifies ableism.

As stigmatized people, mentally disabled people can feel alone, ostracized, and afraid. These feelings create greater struggles, such as a fear of seeking help, a fear of disclosing one's disabilities (leading to masking, which causes psychological damage), and more. If higher education institutions want students to reach out for help when they are in mental health crises, they must work to eradicate mental health stigma on campus. Otherwise, community members will continue to suffer alone for fear of being stigmatized.

Person-First and Identity-First Language

Person-first language is phrasing that puts the person (frequently, literally the word "person") in front of someone's disability, like this: "a person with autism." When first pushed for by disability rights activists in the 1970s, person-first language aimed to end the reduction of a disabled person to their disability: to end the erasing of a disabled person's humanity.[22] Person-first language ended the use of terms like "a schizophrenic" by providing instead "a person with schizophrenia." "A manic-depressive" became "a person with bipolar disorder." These new phrases humanized disabled people.

But today, for many disabled people, it is time to set aside person-first language in favor of language that allows us to claim our disabilities as part of our identities. Identity-first language is language that prioritizes a disabled person's identity, like this: "an autistic person" or "I am autistic" instead of "a person with autism" or "I have autism." We prefer identity-first language because we view our disabilities as a part of us ("am") not something that is appended to us ("with"). For example, I am mentally disabled. I am a mentally disabled person. Thus, I do not like the phrase "a person with mental disabilities" because it shunts my disabilities off to the side, like an accessory or, worse, something I should be ashamed of. I do not carry my disabilities around in my satchel with my laptop or hide them from view.

Autistic advocate Lydia X. Z. Brown points out how many autistic people have embraced identity-first language: "In the autism community, many self-advocates and their allies prefer terminology such as 'Autistic,' 'Autistic person,' or 'Autistic individual' because we understand autism as an inherent part of an individual's identity."[23] I agree. There is no line where my personality ends and my autism begins. I am not "a person with autism" because I do not carry autism around in my satchel.

The phrase "mental illness," however, presents a linguistic challenge: to *have* a mental illness and to *be* mentally ill refer to two different things. Because mental illnesses can be treatable, and because mental illnesses can be dormant and then flare, one could have a mental illness yet not be mentally ill. For example, as I write this, I have bipolar disorder, which is a mental illness, but I am not, at the moment, mentally ill. To put it another way, sometimes because I have bipolar disorder, I am depressed. Sometimes I am manic.

Not every disabled person agrees with the perspective that identity-first language is better than person-first language. There are also many normates who insist that person-first language is better. My only request is this: when you are figuring out how to talk about disabled people, please listen to disabled people about the language they prefer. We should be the ones who decide how we are described.

I'll end with this: the purpose of using identity-first language is to affirm a person's identity as a disabled person, and that is a good thing. Don't stuff our disabilities in a satchel.

Invisible Disabilities

Sometimes a person who appears to be normate is actually disabled, but you can't tell because the disabled person can hide their disabilities. An "invisible disability" is a disability that a disabled person can hide, completely or mostly, in social situations. This ability to hide a disability and blend into normate society is a privilege. When a person hides their mental disabilities, they do what is called "masking," described below.

For example, sometimes I try very hard to appear normate rather than mentally disabled, and frequently I succeed. What usually happens is that normates think I'm quirky: I talk too quickly and more than is appropriate for a given situation; I blurt out the wrong things and struggle with social norms. To outsiders who do not know I am disabled, I can seem over-caffeinated and awkward.

Research has shown that disabled people with invisible disabilities who seek accommodations face a great deal of suspicion and mistrust. Disability legal studies scholar Doron Dorfman, in his empirical research on normates' reactions to disability accommodations, found that "[normate] participants were always much more suspicious of a person with a nonvisible disability" who sought disability resources.[24] In his research, visible disabilities reassured normates that a disabled person wasn't trying to cheat the system. Despite this challenge, having an invisible disability is a privilege because it can allow a person to appear nondisabled and avoid much of the stigma against mental disability.

Masking

One way that a mentally disabled person can make sure their disabilities remain invisible is by "masking." As autistic psychology researcher Hannah Belcher explains, "To 'mask' or to 'camouflage' means to hide or disguise parts of oneself in order to better fit in with those around you."[25] "Masking" is a term that originated to describe the social camouflaging done by autistic people, but other neurodivergent people mask and use the term as well.

Masking is harmful to mentally disabled people. Belcher describes how autistic masking can include "suppressing certain behaviours we find soothing but that others think are 'weird,' such as stimming or intense interests. It can also mean mimicking the behaviour of those around us, such as copying non-verbal behaviours, and developing complex social scripts to get by in social situations." Thus, when a mentally disabled person is masking, they are constantly multitasking, even if the masking is happening unconsciously. This work is exhausting and takes a serious psychological toll.

When I am in social situations that require me to suppress my natural behaviors, such as when I am teaching or in work meetings with acquaintances or strangers, I mask unconsciously. When I am masking, every decision I make runs through the masking test. Are these words okay to speak? Am I reading this person's cues correctly? Was that statement a question that requires an answer? Am I fidgeting too much? Doing all of this unconscious work while also participating in the social activity itself is exhausting. Plus, I constantly worry that if my filter fails, the social backlash may be swift and painful—because in the past, it has been. Now I try to mask less and less, to live my disabilities out loud. But like many fellow disabled people, I have a lifetime of masking habits to unlearn.

The toll masking takes on mentally disabled people, as research shows, goes beyond exhaustion. It can also cause depression, anxiety, and an increased risk of suicide. Research on autistic adults who mask shows that "where camouflaging is unsuccessful, strenuous, or if the person feels forced to camouflage, it may be associated with high stress level, low mood and low self-esteem."[26] When mentally disabled people mask, we hide our true identities and cannot seek acceptance by our friends and family. And, by extension, we cannot learn to accept ourselves.

Masking and other protective measures feel necessary because of the negative stereotypes attached to mental disability—and all disabilities. For example, media portrayals of "disability fakers" have negatively influenced public opinion about disabled people seeking accommodations and social security benefits. Dorfman gives examples of negative media headlines, such as "'Disability Act Abused? Law's Use Sparks Debate' or 'The Disabilities Act's Parade of Absurdities.'"[27] These media portrayals have a material effect on disabled people, because, as Dorfman explains, they can "shape how people experience their rights, how they are willing to exercise them, and how the law itself is being shaped to respond to this suspicion."[28] These suspicions quite literally shape the laws that affect disabled people.

If we, as a society, talk about mentally disabled people in ways that stereotype, scapegoat, and shame, we create an environment in which mentally disabled people must keep their disabilities secret, avoid medical help, and, when facing struggles, struggle alone. We must combat these negative stereotypes by using language of inclusivity, as I have presented here, and create communities in which mentally disabled people are embraced and can unmask.

Accommodations vs. Accessibility

Although the terms "accommodations" and "accessibility" are often used interchangeably, they do not mean the same thing. In fact, in my work I've argued that they are diametrically opposed. Accommodations are special exceptions made for one particular disabled person. They require a person to jump through lots of administrative hoops and give up their privacy to get them. They are frequently expensive. Accommodations frame disability as an institutional annoyance and burden, something outside the mainstream, a bump in an institution's otherwise smooth road. And, if one believes accommodations are a burden, it is easy to infer that disabled people are a burden.

Why are accommodations needed at all? Institutions frequently blame disabled people for needing them. But that blame is misplaced; our society has created the burden by ignoring the existence of disabled people. Accommodations are necessary because we, as a society, create spaces that are inaccessible to disabled people.[29] And then, when disabled people need access to certain spaces, we, as a society, are forced to make special accommodations so they can access those spaces. The key word is "special": accommodations are always special, extra, more. And anything extra or special is a burden.

When disabled students need accommodations, many faculty and administrators believe the students have created a burden on an institution, on a professor, or on their fellow students. Disabled students know that many people feel this way; that is why many never request accommodations in the first place. In a 2017 study of autistic college students, only 65 percent of them registered with disability services.[30] Of those, only 68 percent who received accommodations reported that the accommodations met their needs. Worse, "even among the participants who reported that the accommodations met expectations, several

reported some difficulties with either the process or with professor adherence." One student reported that "it was absolute hell trying to get
them [professors] to understand that the accommodations are necessary." Another student reported, "Sometimes the professor does not
comply and there is nothing that can be done."

Most people do not question the accommodations model of disability
support, believing, falsely, "Hasn't it always been this way?" or "This is
the only way it can possibly be." Our current onerous accommodations
model is not the way it has always been, and it is certainly *not* the way it
must be. In the first place, getting accommodations does not need to be
so onerous (as I describe in Chapter 5).

More importantly, providing accommodations is not the only way to
make space for disabled people in our communities. There is also accessibility. In the disability context, I define accessibility as the existence of
a space that is hospitable to and usable by all disabled people, always,
all the time. As I wrote in 2017: "Accommodation is not accessibility. If
a space is accessible, that space is always, 100% of the time, welcoming
to disabled people. Disabled people do not have to ask for anything.
They do not have to prove they have disabilities. They do not have to
interact with gatekeepers. They can simply be."[31] The accommodations
model treats disabled people as unexpected outliers. Accessibility treats
disabled people as an expected part of a community.

Accessibility shifts the burden from disabled people onto institutions, where it belongs. Institutions should be the ones shouldering the
burden of disability access, not individuals, because institutions have a
duty to account for their entire community, not just for normates. Accessibility is not a necessary evil or a bump in the road. It does not force
disabled people to disclose our disabilities to strangers, which is an invasion of privacy that our society has come to accept as normal. Indeed,
the accommodations model works only if it can invade the privacy of
disabled people. Accessibility, on the other hand, allows disabled people
to choose to whom to disclose their disabilities.

Better still, accessibility is not just for those who have diagnosed disabilities. It is for those of us who are undiagnosed. I wasn't diagnosed
with bipolar disorder until I finished college, and my autism diagnosis came decades later. But my mental disabilities affected, sometimes
greatly, my ability to succeed in school.

One way to think about accommodations and accessibility is with the concepts of exclusion and inclusion. Accommodations are based on the premise that disabled people are *excluded* as a natural state of affairs. Therefore, to include an individual disabled person, an institution must make unique, individual changes for that person. Accessibility is premised on *inclusion*, that disabled people are part of a community, and, therefore, every resource that community has to offer is available to them as a matter of course.

Teaching Through Liberatory Language

As professors, we must incorporate inclusive and liberatory disability language into our teaching. Our words have the power to shape the world our students and colleagues live in. Avoid using "schizo," "bipolar," or "OCD" as metaphors—all you have to do is find better metaphors. That's an easy win.

Eradicating the ableism that has wormed its way into our everyday language is hard but necessary work. This chapter provides a starting point for doing so. College is a time when students are at great risk for developing mental health struggles and mental disabilities. Using language to create an environment where they feel safe seeking help for those struggles should be a priority for all of us.

Part I

The Mental Health Crisis in Higher Education

1

Anxiety in Academia

I can't remember a time when I didn't worry endlessly. Even as a child I was anxious. (It turns out that anxiety correlates with autism.[1] Of course, we didn't know I was autistic back then.)

Anxiety dogged me through college, when I constantly worried that I wore the wrong clothes or said the wrong words or majored in the wrong thing. It was a rare moment when I felt safe in my choices. Anxiety felt like an itching all over my body, like my skin was too tight. I would have horrible nightmares, and then I wouldn't sleep at all. To soothe myself, I would try to control things: writing a paper early, for example, so I wouldn't have to worry about the assignment hanging over my head like the mythical sword. Friends thought I was just a fast writer. No—I was a worried one.

In law school, though, it wasn't possible to work ahead fast enough to soothe my anxiety—that's not how law school is designed. I started drinking too much in an attempt to tamp down the itching, the worrying, the unbearable feeling of my world spinning out of control. Luckily, I found a psychiatrist who helped me stop drinking before I spun out entirely. She helped me through graduate school, where I was able to focus and remain far steadier.

Now, years later, I have good anxiety medicine, and it helps, mostly. As I write this book, occasionally the itching, squeezing, am-I-going-to-die feeling kicks in, and I have to take a miraculous pill and lie down for a while. My anxieties about the book are endless because I worry it won't do all of the things that I need it to do—and that is a long list. Mostly I worry that I won't be able to convince you, dear reader, to care enough about mental disability to help me change the world.

And the fact is, I can't control your reactions to my words. Indeed, in this life, there isn't much we can control at all. But if you have anxiety, you don't have a choice but to try. And if you are in higher education, faculty or student, you are likely trying very, very hard.

Anxiety Haunts Higher Education

In a 2018 study, 39 percent of faculty and staff reported having some type of anxiety, along with 42 percent of students.[2] Compare these numbers with the general US population, which, according to the National Institute of Mental Health, is 19 percent in a given year.[3]

Why does anxiety spike in the ivory tower?

When it comes to mental disability, it is easy to blame the individual for their symptoms or diagnosis. But a systemic rise of anxiety disorders in higher education is caused by systemic problems, not individual "weakness." Take, for example, the structural inequities faced by contingent faculty. Contingent faculty, and the inequities they face, have been on the rise for decades as institutions have sought ways to cut costs by cutting the faculty payroll. Claire Bond Potter, history professor and longtime higher education critic, writes that institutions use the "illusion that contingent labor is a kind of piggy bank that can be raided when universities want to build new institutes, recruit star faculty, and expand their campuses."[4] For decades now, colleges have sought to recruit students by building climbing walls and high-end dorms, and a lot of that money has come from cutting full-time faculty jobs. More and more teaching is now done by professors working contingent positions—adjuncts, visitors, short-term lecturers, and the like.

Now colleges are reaping what they sowed. They face labor organizing and strikes as contingent professors are no longer willing to put up with terrible wages and working conditions.[5] They also face the negative effects of these terrible working conditions on contingent faculty, who now teach over 70 percent of undergraduate courses. Psychology research shows that these professors experience greater stress, anxiety, and depression because of their insecure employment.[6]

The anxiety experienced by contingent faculty is just one example of how structural problems of higher education create conditions that cause mental disabilities. Others include the immense pressure certain faculty feel to perform under onerous conditions, such as those I call "front-line faculty." Front-line faculty do more than their fair share of the emotional carework of students because of their job positions or marginalized status in the university. Contingent professors are front-line faculty because they frequently have a lot of one-on-one student contact and can't opt out because of their job insecurity. People of color are also front-line faculty. If you are the only Black faculty member in your department, you will find yourself, by default, responsible for the well-being of all Black students in your department. (Chapter 13 addresses front-line faculty in great detail.)

When we teach, we must presume that any student we are teaching is dealing with anxiety. If 42 percent of students have anxiety, then we're just playing the odds. These high student numbers also mean that many of our students are facing anxiety for the first time. Anxiety is yet another new challenge in the midst of all the others that college is handing them. The prevalence of anxiety in higher education makes it imperative that we all understand more about anxiety disorders and how they affect our colleagues and students.

These high rates of anxiety among our students and colleagues often mean that anxiety disappears as background noise in academia. We just say we're "stressed out" and roll with it. Like any systemic problem, maintaining focus on the epidemic of anxiety in higher education is a challenge. When a problem is everywhere, it can appear to be nowhere. When a problem becomes prevalent, it stops being a problem and starts being the norm. We cannot allow the debilitating anxiety among faculty and students to become a norm that we accept simply because it is prevalent.

The normalization of suffering is the trap of systemic burnout, anxiety, depression, and other common mental disabilities in higher education. Systemic mental health struggles become hard to notice even when they are in our classrooms, in our advising offices, in our libraries, and among our colleagues. Anxiety has become a hard-to-spot campus crisis. Faculty and students are manifesting anxiety all around us, and it is our collective duty to notice it and to do something about it.

Not Just Overblown Worry

Anxiety disorders can seem, to those who do not understand it, like a small thing—just overblown worry. To anxiety outsiders, it can seem that a person with an anxiety disorder is unable to control something that should be easily controlled. They are just too weak to get a grip on ordinary fears. These outsiders are wrong. But what, exactly, are anxiety disorders?

According to clinical psychologist Owen Kelly, "Anxiety disorders are serious mental illnesses that cause significant worry or fear that doesn't go away and may even get worse over time."[7] "Anxiety" refers to a group of disorders—not just one thing—each with its own sources and symptoms. Furthermore, each person's experience of anxiety is unique. Anxiety disorders include generalized anxiety disorder, panic disorder (which leads to panic attacks), obsessive-compulsive disorder (OCD), and more.

Generalized anxiety disorder (GAD) is the medical diagnosis most laypeople refer to when they say "anxiety" or "anxiety disorder." It has three diagnostic criteria in the American Psychiatric Association's *Diagnostic and Statistical Manual of Mental Disorders* (DSM):

(1) A person feels "excessive anxiety and worry (apprehensive expectation), occurring more days than not for at least 6 months, about a number of events or activities (such as work or school performance)."

(2) It is "difficult to control the worry."

(3) The anxiety is associated with three or more of the six symptoms the DSM lists with the criteria.[8] Here are the six symptoms: (a) "Restlessness or feeling keyed up or on edge," (b) "Being easily fatigued," (c) "Difficulty concentrating or mind going blank," (d) "Irritability," (e) "Muscle tension," and (f) "Sleep disturbance."[9]

Let's look at some of the key words in this criteria list. The worry is "excessive." It is "about a number of events." It is "difficult to control." What these words tell us is that anxiety is not focused on a single point in time or a single event, and, furthermore, it isn't something a person can wrestle into obedience. One can rarely, if ever, beat anxiety by toughing it out. The entire point is that it is difficult to control.

Then there are the impairments that anxiety creates: restlessness and difficulty concentrating, for example. A person feels fatigue yet has difficulty sleeping, which is incredibly frustrating. A person feels ongoing irritability and tension. Imagine trying to work under these conditions, whether as faculty or a student.

I interviewed a colleague, Sarah (a pseudonym), a professor at a large, R1 state university.[10] Sarah attended an Ivy League graduate program, one of the very top in her field, and she teaches primarily graduate students. As a professor, she conducts herself professionally, and her students adore her. Yet, despite all of her achievements, Sarah deals with chronic anxiety. She explained to me how chronic anxiety affects her on a daily basis at work: "What chronic anxiety means in the context of my job is that I am constantly worrying, second-guessing myself, or catastrophizing. It means that I hold myself to impossible standards and, when I predictably fail to meet them, conclude that I am worthless."

She also pointed out the connection between her contingent faculty job and anxiety: "The intersection of being a contingent faculty member and having anxiety is a tough place to be," she told me. In particular, her position means, "I question every interaction with other faculty and with administration. For example, I write my annual self-evaluation and then, after submitting it, keep rereading it to figure out whether I said anything inappropriate." Sarah's experience with anxiety in higher education is not an outlier. In my research, I have discovered that Sarah is the norm.

The Illusion of Control

At the heart of anxiety is the need to feel control over one's environment. Sometimes you make decisions based on a psychological need to stop feeling out of control—even if you do not realize that you are doing so. You might make decisions too quickly—"snap" decisions—in order to pull yourself out of uncomfortable limbo. Control, and the power of your snap decision to give it to you, is, of course, an illusion. But waiting in limbo can feel so unsettling that any decision is better than none. Later, you might regret the snap decision that you made. Say you are looking for a new teaching position. You apply for three. You really want Position One. But you are so worried about getting a job at all that when your least favorite job offer comes in first, you accept it right away. You immediately feel relief that you have a new position. But that relief is short-lived. Should you have asked for more time to consider the first offer you received? Could you have used that time to reach out to Position One to see if you were being considered for the job? Probably. Instead, you snatched up the first job offer you received because you felt so uncomfortable waiting in job-hunt limbo and wanted to seize control of the situation. Anxiety makes it difficult or impossible to sit in limbo.

Sarah described to me how anxiety and the need for control manifests when it is time to grade her students' final papers. She told me, "Memories of how important grades can be, combined with the difficulty I have trusting my own judgment, my anxiety-driven perfectionism, the value I place on my relationships with students, and a mandatory curve [required by her school] means that grading is torture for me." All of these elements of grading cause Sarah to feel that grading is out of her control, spiking her anxiety. So she tries to regain that control with anxiety-driven behaviors: "I read and reread and reread each paper individually and in combination with others, and then I question my own judgment about what I just read." The obsessive rereading is an attempt to wrestle the grading process under control—perhaps on the *next* reread, Sarah thinks, grading will make sense, will be easy, will no longer make her feel like she is failing at her job. (It doesn't.) The rereading of the papers is an attempt to exert control over the anxiety-producing grading process.

Worse, she told me, "as I'm reading the papers, I decide that all [student] mistakes are attributable to me because I should have done a better job teaching and communicating concepts." She's wrong, of course, but the self-blame, ironically, is another way of soothing her anxiety by exerting control. If Sarah blames herself for her students' less-than-stellar performance, then, anxiety-logic says, she can control the outcome of her students' learning.

Catastrophizing: "What If ... ?"

Catastrophizing is focusing on a specific worry to the point that you turn it into a horrible disaster in your mind. In psychology terms, catastrophizing is "the process by which worriers perceive progressively worse and worse outcomes to a specific worry topic."[11] Catastrophizing "is usually the result of the worrier posing automatic questions of the 'what if . . . ?' kind." When anxiety causes you to catastrophize, down the rabbit hole goes your brain, taking what is, in the end, an ordinary setback and turning it into a nightmare.

Sarah described to me how she catastrophizes after turning in her grades. There is always a student (or two) whose grades she particularly agonized over. After she turns in grades, she told me, "for the next week or two, that student's name follows me around. I think about it in the shower, when I'm playing with my kids, when I'm driving in the car, when I'm trying to do other work. I think about their name and then feel doubt, guilt, shame." All of these horrible feelings build up to a catastrophizing moment: "I tell myself, 'I'm a terrible professor. What am I doing if I can't do this part of the job? They're going to hate me. I should have read their paper again. I'm lazy. I'm a terrible person.'" Of course, Sarah is none of those things. But anxiety disorders do not care about the truth. Her brain takes a specific worry—that she might have given a student an unfair grade (she didn't)—and runs with it, creating a catastrophe, specifically, that Sarah is not only a terrible professor, but a terrible person too.

Rumination: "If I Had Just . . . "

Rumination is a manifestation of anxiety "that involves repetitively and passively focusing on symptoms of distress and on the possible causes and consequences of these symptoms."[12] Rumination is focused on the *past*, on something that has gone wrong. Instead of accepting the past event and moving on, the ruminator wants to fix what has gone wrong—a form of exerting control, the hallmark of anxiety. People with anxiety ruminate "because they mistakenly believe they could have controlled or changed" a past outcome they believe to be negative.[13] Of course, it is impossible to fix something that has already gone wrong. But anxiety doesn't care about the impossible.

They—or I should say *we*—frequently experience this particular manifestation of anxiety as a repetitive thought process that goes like this: "If I had just . . . , If I had just . . . ," and on and on, fixated on the past disaster and how we could have avoided it. But all that thinking about past events and how to control them only makes things worse: "Rumination does not lead to active problem solving to change circumstances."[14] Rather, "people who are ruminating remain fixated on the problems and on their feelings about them without taking action." Because we're stuck in the past, we can't make actual plans for the future.

Rumination often stems from perfectionism. When we fail to live up to our own high standards, we ruminate on our perceived failures. (I talk more about perfectionism and failure in Chapter 4, "Toxic Academic

Overwork.") Sarah gave me an example of how she ruminates over her teaching, driven by perfectionism: "Sometimes I have to meet with students as they prepare to write their final (graded) projects. I dread these meetings because the stakes feel so high. When the meetings are over, I think about whether my answers to their questions were perfect." Of course, her answers weren't perfect—nothing ever is. But her anxiety takes that lack of perfection and ruminates: "I replay the meetings over and over and decide I've said something misleading or problematic or I've led my students astray in some fashion." She is unable to set aside past events and accept she did the best job she could, which is, in reality, a very good job. But anxiety takes a smallish thing and turns it into a monster.

Rumination does not actually care about a solution to a problem. Despite all of the energy a ruminator spends thinking about whatever causes the distress, rumination never makes things better. It's an anxiety trap that can feel impossible to escape from.

Anxiety and Procrastination

For faculty and students alike, one of the terrible outcomes of anxiety can be procrastination. Procrastination is not laziness. As psychologist Devon Price has famously written, "laziness does not exist."[15] Procrastination, according to Price, is driven either by anxiety or by a lack of understanding of the task. Price points out that procrastination is actually more likely to occur when a person cares more about a task rather than less, which causes them to become paralyzed by fear of failure. (I delve deeper into procrastination in Chapter 14, "Procrastination and Compassion.")

Sarah explained to me how anxiety and procrastination work together to get in the way of her scholarship: "My anxiety impedes my scholarly productivity. I am convinced that I can't possibly have anything worthwhile to say. Once I have an idea, I procrastinate. I'm daunted by the task—a task I know I am theoretically capable of, but which seems daunting and insurmountable." Why does it seem insurmountable? Anxiety convinces Sarah that because her work is less than perfect, she shouldn't bother with it. She explained, "What could I possibly have to contribute to any ongoing conversation? Why is it worth doing if it isn't groundbreaking and perfect? It's not—and perfect is too much to ask for, so I remain daunted and quiet." Sarah's experience is a classic demonstration of the relationship between anxiety and procrastination, driven by perfectionism, one that many of our colleagues—and students—struggle with.

A main cause of procrastination, essentially, is the belief that you are terrible at what you do—as Sarah puts it, "What could I possibly have to contribute?" The answer that goes unspoken is "nothing."[16] A procrastinator frequently believes they have nothing important to say because they, themselves, are not important. Procrastination is deeply linked with anxiety and depression, and it derives from negative feelings about oneself.

If you have a student or colleague spiraling with anxiety and procrastination, you should intervene. However, you should not intervene with punishment—say, a nasty email about how your colleague isn't pulling their weight on a committee—but with compassion. When a colleague (or student) is failing to turn in work on time, let's jump to the conclusion that they are running off the rails, rather than being lazy. Let's conclude that they need help. We want our colleagues and students to be healthy and to succeed. We do not want them to wash out. (If you don't mind your colleagues and students washing out, you should probably stop reading this book now.)

Approaching our colleague (or student) with compassion and encouraging them to feel self-compassion is the best way to help them get back on track and complete the work they need to—and *want* to—complete. No one knows more than they do that they've fallen behind. And no one wants to fix that problem more. If you show them compassion and help them find compassion for themselves, you are far more likely to get the results you both want.

Anxiety has become so prevalent on campus that it has become hard to spot. Nevertheless, we must all be vigilant. If you are struggling with anxiety, you need to seek help. If you see yourself reflected in this chapter, talk to someone who will help you manage your anxiety. If you see a colleague who is struggling, offer to help them find resources. Living with anxiety can be hell. No one should have to.

2

Population Shock Events

When I was a law student at the University of North Carolina, in the law school building was a large basement social space we called "The Rumpus Room" (really). Sofas were scattered about the room, and a large television that was almost always tuned into sports.

Early in the morning of September 11, 2001, I was a first-year law student heading to class, still half asleep, when my dear friend L. grabbed me by the arm and dragged me down the stairs to The Rumpus Room. Crammed in the room with a hundred of my fellow law students, I watched the Twin Towers fall.

Days and weeks later, the initial panic abated. We were finally able to reach friends and family by phone after the massive disruption of cell service was over. We knew who had lived and who had died. But for weeks and months after 9/11, the trauma did not end. Our school community was in a collective daze—and North Carolina is nowhere near Ground Zero.

What my fellow students and I experienced back in 2001, along with so many others around the country and the world, can be described as a "population shock event."[1] Population shock events are large-scale social disruptions.[2] They are "unexpected or unpredictable events that disrupt the environmental, health, economic, or social circumstances within a population."[3] Research shows that this sort of disruption "can increase the prevalence of depressive and anxiety disorders." Researchers have been using this concept as a way to understand the long-term effects of the COVID-19 pandemic on mental health.

As the example of 9/11 illustrates, population shock events occurred long before the pandemic. These shock events leave powerful wakes, affect many people for a long time, and give no time to regroup because the trauma compounds rather than dissipates. For example, after 9/11, the US government instituted many rapid changes that kept Americans on edge: new airport screenings, the creation of the Department of Homeland Security, a color-coded terror alert system, and a decades-long war. Although the 9/11 attacks were a massive shock event, they left a compounding traumatic wake.

In higher education we have our own particular shock events. Mass shootings on campuses, tragedies that occur far too frequently, cause ripple effects at institutions around the nation. In some schools, students and faculty must do active shooter drills, many of which are traumatizing in their own right.[4] (Some school trainings use foam projectiles to mimic real guns, a traumatic experience I cannot imagine putting students through.[5])

Past shock events have taught us a lot about the COVID shock event. Joshua A. Gordon, the director of the National Institute of Mental Health, wrote that "much of what we have learned from past disasters and epidemics is holding true in the context of the COVID-19 pandemic."[6] That is, with COVID, as with past shock events, there have been "substantial increases in self-reported behavioral health symptoms." But, Gordon notes, the COVID-19 pandemic differs from these previous shock events: "Unlike other population shocks, COVID-19 has become global, disrupting many aspects of life for most, if not all, of the world's populations." It is fair to say, then, that the COVID-19 pandemic is the most widespread population shock event most of us have ever experienced, faculty and students alike. Its effects are truly worldwide. And although COVID has affected different populations in different ways, it has affected nearly everyone.

We can learn a lot from the COVID-19 pandemic about how the trauma of a population shock event affects collective mental health, particularly in the context of higher education—knowledge that we can take with us into the future.

Population Shock Events and Mental Health Trauma

Living with a population shock event causes mental health trauma. When I use the term "mental health trauma," I mean long-lasting harm to a person's mental health. And that is what we are seeing all around us post-COVID (if, indeed, we are post-COVID)—mental health trauma on a mass scale. After years of immense strain, nearly everyone is on the ropes, whether they wish to acknowledge it or not. Studies from the CDC, National Institute of Mental Health, and more have shown that mental illness has risen to crisis levels.[7] For example, a *Lancet* study found that anxiety disorder and depression diagnoses in the United States post-pandemic are up more than 25 percent.[8] That news is bad enough; for those of us in higher education, however, the news is even worse. The age group most affected by the rise in anxiety disorders and depression are those aged 20–24. That is, the age group that encompasses many, if not most, of our students.

Psychologists have another term to describe shock events: "collective trauma." Psychologist Gilad Hirschberger explains, "Collective trauma . . . constitutes a cataclysmic event that affects not only direct victims, but society as a whole."[9] These cataclysmic events are, Hirschberger notes, "devastating for individuals and for groups."[10] Faculty development professional and neurodiversity expert Karen Ray Costa, who has ADHD, gives examples of collective trauma in her work, including, "the scourges of racism, sexism, ableism, and other forms of oppression are absolutely examples of collective traumas," as are "gun violence and natural disasters . . . [which] have had both direct and indirect impacts on college campuses."[11] Costa notes that "the darkest days of traumas, generally speaking, fall well after the impact. I fear that people don't realize that the hard part often begins when the traumatic event is over." As Costa points out, the notion that because the "shock" is over we can move on is wrong-headed. The pain of a population shock/collective trauma does not simply end when the shock ends. It compounds, causing mental and physical harm to individuals, until it is properly addressed through a "reconstruction" process requiring grief and healing.

In higher education, the collective trauma of the pandemic went beyond the medical, beyond the virus. COVID closed our institutions' doors in a rush in March of 2020, shocking us all. It kept them closed for at least a year, forcing faculty and students into a new and frequently uncomfortable learning environment. It then created a difficult, sometimes ugly debate about reopening, which in turn created painful conflict between professors, students, and administration.

In the fall of 2021, my institution resumed teaching in person. During the first few months back on campus, my colleagues and I persistently worried about our health and the health of our families due to our exposure at work. I taught my seminar in a classroom that had plenty of seating for the number of students, but that was, nevertheless, small. I am lucky that my students were very compliant with wearing masks, but I frequently felt unsafely close to them.

I interviewed a professor who teaches at a medium-sized private university in the South.[12] She told me that, during that same school year, she struggled with students who did not comply with her institution's COVID policies. As a contingent faculty member, she did not know what to do if a student did not wipe down their desk before and after class, or if a student did not keep on their mask. "The dynamic of having to enforce [COVID] rules rather than teaching my course put a terrible strain on my relationship with my students." She notes that her experience points to bigger structural issues about precarity and how contingent faculty are not supported by their institutions. I can see her point: when your job depends on positive course evaluations, you do not want to hassle your students about masks. She told me, "They [the institution] basically passed off the responsibility onto us. . . . I felt really responsible for my students' health."

COVID health policies were a new, necessary burden, but the old burdens remained—contingency, for example—and frequently loomed larger than before, as this interview shows. Like many of us, I spent the first weeks and months back at work slogging through a backlog while also managing an environment that kept throwing new, unpredictable institutional challenges my way—such as students in dire need of mental health support. The stress of the pandemic shock event continues to take a toll on the mental health of both faculty and students. In the classroom, students continue to express their mental health struggles by turning in late assignments, being absent from class, and dropping out altogether.

As Costa points out, "Lasting impacts [of the COVID collective trauma] are immense and probably just beginning. To deny this denies reality."[13] She writes that COVID has "shattered" us; now we must do the work of "putting [ourselves] back together again."

Mental Disability, Population Shock, and Higher Education

Predictably, COVID-19 stressors hit disabled people even harder than they did normates (nondisabled people). Stress researchers describe how "shared traumatic events" harm disabled people via a cycle called "macro-level stress proliferation."[14] This cycle of stress proliferation has two steps. First, a shared traumatic event "spur[s] a number of individual-level stressors" for a disabled person, which can also lead to a worsening of the person's disability. For a mentally disabled person in higher education, these individual-level stressors might include the loss of accommodations, difficulty using new, mandatory technology, loss of necessary campus support systems due to isolation, loss of medical care, and heightened loneliness, depression, and anxiety. In short, the first part of the cycle makes the lives of mentally disabled faculty and students much worse.

Next, these individual-level stressors make it harder for a disabled person to respond to the macro-level event—the shock event. For example, without access to accommodations, medical care, or other necessary things, a mentally disabled person cannot do their work as well. If a disabled person cannot do their work, they might lose their job or get kicked out of school. In short, mentally disabled people, and all disabled people, get hit harder by shock events than normates do, causing greater strain on each individual disabled person. This strain, in turn, makes it more difficult for a disabled person to respond to the shock event. Then the cycle begins again.

Here's an example. Healthcare resources for mentally disabled people have always been difficult to come by, but the pandemic has made this scarce resource even scarcer. According to the *Journal of the American Medical Association*, during COVID, "about 45% of the US population [is] living in an area with a shortage of mental health professionals, particularly in rural areas."[15] In December of 2021, my therapist told me she was leaving her practice, giving me only two weeks' notice and no plan for continuing my care. I felt grief because I was losing this relationship, anger because she left so abruptly, and fear because I no longer had care. I called her former practice and asked to be put on the waitlist for a new therapist. They told me it would be months before another therapist had an opening. Mental health care for a person with mental disabilities is not optional, but during a shock event care can be hard to come by.

Without care, dealing with the shock event is harder. What I have described is a structural problem, not a personal one; however, for a mentally disabled person, the structural problem has personal consequences.

Similarly, there is a perennial shortage of mental health care on campus, now exacerbated because of the shock event. Institutions are strapped for funds (because COVID caused enrollments to drop), and mental health care providers are in great demand (also because of COVID). Therefore, mentally disabled students and students struggling with their mental health frequently do not have the care they need. The stress that mentally disabled students and faculty have experienced during the pandemic proliferates from the public to the private, the macro to the micro, and then back again, until our resources are depleted.

Burgeoning Mental Disability

The pandemic has caused widespread mental health trauma, including spikes in rates of depression and anxiety. This widespread mental health trauma will cause many people to develop mental disabilities. Some of these new diagnoses will be long lasting. That is, some of the people—our own colleagues and students—diagnosed with an anxiety disorder or depression will develop a permanent mental disability.

However, these newly disabled colleagues and students may not choose to identify as such. Moving from a normate identity to a disabled identity is a huge shift. Calling yourself disabled is, in part, a risky political act. Although there is power that comes with claiming a disabled identity, there is also great vulnerability—especially in higher education—because of the stigma against mental disability.

If you are a faculty member who has developed anxiety or depression or another mental disability under COVID, you have many reasons to keep your mental disability secret from your colleagues. Stigma in higher education causes the widespread belief that to be mentally disabled means to be broken and wrong. Stigma creates negative stereotyping and isolation of mentally disabled people. Stigma also works internally on disabled people themselves, creating feelings of isolation and shame. If you are mentally disabled in higher education, you are in a double bind: suffer in private alone or reach out for help and risk ostracization.

Disabled people, like other marginalized people, are the first to suffer and suffer worse during times of societal stress. But because we are suffering, we also tend to be the first to notice that others are suffering, and we support one another. In higher education, we are often beacons to others who are newly suffering, welcoming them, often in secret, to give them help and advice as they confront disabilities for the first time. But giving this help and advice to our colleagues and students creates extra labor for disabled faculty. However, we do it anyway because we are the only ones our newly mentally disabled community members feel safe talking to.

There are so many ways that the mental health trauma caused by the pandemic can manifest: burnout, depression, anxiety, and so on. But it is also important to note that these mental health struggles and mental disabilities in higher education are not new—higher education faced a mental health crisis long before COVID. The pandemic exacerbated the crisis and brought it into the national conversation. We must use the attention that COVID has caused institutions to give to mental health on campus to make changes for the better.

After any shock event, there is no going back. There is only forward, and ideally forward for the better. As disabled author and activist Alice Wong writes, "The whole pressure to return to what we think of as [pre-COVID] normal is something we need to let go. I want everyone to think about looking ahead as a real chance to rethink the world."[16] Costa points out that the social pressures to return to some imagined normal after a collective trauma are inappropriate if not impossible.[17] She writes, "Higher ed will not be the higher ed that it was before." Post-COVID, higher education must, according to Costa, "[open] itself up to the possibility of a new higher ed, a more humane, loving, hopeful higher ed." What might that look like?

Campus communities must work toward normalizing and destigmatizing mental disabilities and mental health struggles. When this stigma is lessened, community members will feel less ashamed seeking help when they are in crisis. To break down stigma, communities must start with how they treat their mentally disabled students and faculty. How accessible are learning and working environments? Is there a culture of overwork that harms mentally disabled people and pushes them out of higher education altogether? If we are inclusive of mental disabilities, we can create a truly neurodiverse community.

3

Systemic Burnout

It is midmorning, and I am sitting in the digital waiting room to meet with my therapist. On my phone, a text message comes in from a colleague. She lives in another state, but she is someone I speak with regularly, and she has been going through a very hard time lately.

The text message reads: *I'm driving. Please. Call me if you have time to talk.*

The word "please"—complete with a punctuation mark—causes me to feel a sting of worry. I call her immediately, even as my therapist is dialing into the teleconference. When my therapist's face appears on the screen, I hold up a finger to her, silently asking her to wait.

While I wait for my friend to answer her phone, I nervously pace around my home office. Finally, she answers.

"Are you okay?" I immediately ask her.

"Oh, yes. I'm okay," she says. "I just had some time to talk while I'm driving."

I explain that I was worried because of her text message. She explains that the odd phrasing and punctuation was due to her use of voice texting.

I think, *That makes sense.*

But the thing is, the week before, this friend was very much not okay—as not-okay as one can be. Her parent recently died, and she was in a very dark place. So it was logical for me to think that something might be off today. I was so attuned to my friend being at risk that all it took for an emergency to register was a single word: "please." And the more I think about it, I wonder whether the "please" was no accident at all.

This friend and I have many mental disabilities between us: bipolar disorder, depression, anxiety, autism. As higher education faculty, we have more education than most people and better access to mental health care too.

But I wonder how the shock of the pandemic has changed us in ways that we may not have realized. Large, traumatic events transform our lives in persistent, rather than transient, ways. Long-term, widespread mental health consequences happen in the years after a traumatic event, in the time when many expect life to have returned to normal.

Because, in the end, this is our normal now.

What Is Burnout?

Higher education has never had a great track record for addressing mental health struggles of students or faculty. Faculty burnout has been an ongoing problem because "we are trained to resist any visible sign of weakness," as burnout expert Rebecca Pope-Ruark explains.[1] Worse, Pope-Ruark writes, faculty wear the notion (if not the reality) of burnout "as a badge of honor" and worship "the cult of busyness that has cursed so many of us to fetishize productivity and reputation." Per Pope-Ruark, this busyness problem is institutional, rooted in "the systematic structures" of academia itself. It was inevitable, then, that faculty would tip into burnout long before the COVID-19 pandemic. COVID merely shined a brighter light on what was already a problem in higher education.

Burnout, as a diagnosis, gained official recognition in 2019, when it was recognized by the International Classification of Diseases, 11th edition (ICD-11), published by the World Health Organization. The ICD-11 defines burnout as "a syndrome conceptualized as resulting from chronic workplace stress that has not been successfully managed."[2] It divides burnout into three "dimensions": (1) "feelings of energy depletion or exhaustion," (2) "increased mental distance from one's job, or feelings of negativism or cynicism related to one's job," and (3) "reduced professional efficacy." The ICD-11 limits burnout, however, to the workplace: "Burn-out refers specifically to phenomena in the occupational context and should not be applied to describe experiences in other areas of life."

Nearly twenty-five years ago, foundational burnout researcher

Christina Maslach and her team defined burnout as "a psychological syndrome in response to chronic interpersonal stressors on the job."[3] Thus, they defined burnout as solely work-related, and the three key dimensions of burnout she and her team identified are the ones the ICD-11 definition is based on. Maslach and her team observed these key causes of burnout: (1) overload (too much work), (2) lack of autonomy, (3) lack of social support, (4) unfair or inequitable treatment, including pay, and (5) lack of reciprocity between worker and employer (again, including pay).

When I first encountered the term "burnout" years ago, it seemed trivial and overused, especially as someone who lives with a "serious" diagnosis like bipolar disorder. As a person with a major mental illness, burnout seemed small and even silly. Maslach and her team point out burnout's poor reputation, writing that it was "derided at first as non-scholarly 'pop psychology.'"[4] To me, it was a fake syndrome invented for investment bankers who had to pull too many hours in order to afford their Maseratis.

I was wrong.

The ironic part of my rejection of burnout was that, ten years ago, I myself experienced career burnout—but did not recognize it at the time. I had spent over a decade working full-time, contingent faculty jobs. Like most of these jobs, which are now endemic to higher education, they had no meaningful advancement, inequitable salaries, and no job security beyond the duration of my contract—and even the contracts felt shaky.

In higher education today, nearly 75 percent of courses are taught by professors with contingent jobs.[5] Furthermore, contingent faculty are "disproportionately female and are more likely than tenured or tenure-track faculty to be Black/African American, Hispanic/Latino, or American Indian than to be Asian or White."[6] Contingent faculty are underpaid, overworked, and undervalued labor who help institutions meet their budgets. As a result of our job status, psychological research has shown that contingent faculty struggle with greater workplace stress, anxiety, and depression.[7] Indeed, the researchers' description of their findings reads like a formula for burnout: "[Contingent] faculty in our sample also identified heavy workload, lack of institutional support such as access to a physical office, and low pay or pay inequity as significant sources of stress." With heavy workloads, lack of institutional support, low pay, and inequitable treatment, it is no wonder that contingent faculty end up burned out, anxious, and depressed.

As a result of these institutional factors, in 2014, I quit my full-time faculty job with barely a plan in place for my next career move. When I quit, I was in full burnout. I was detached and cynical; I had lost any feelings of efficacy and accomplishment with which I had entered the academy. Indeed, I felt like a failure. After I left, I descended into a deep depression, the most dangerous one of my life, which led to a brush with suicide. "Depression and anxiety often accompany burnout," as Pope-Ruark points out.[8] Furthermore, she notes, "if left unchecked burnout can lead to fatigue and sleeplessness, drug and alcohol abuse, and physical health problems, including diabetes, high blood pressure, and heart disease." Burnout is not a fake syndrome; it is real, and it is deadly.

Burnout on the Home Front

Despite the insistence by Maslach and the ICD-11 that burnout must be a workplace phenomenon, the pandemic has revealed that burnout is not, and never has been, a strictly job-related syndrome. The ongoing reality that burnout studies have overlooked up until now is this: burnout encompasses the whole person, both work and home. Spurred by the pandemic, new research on burnout looks at how burnout "spills over" from the workplace to the home and back again.[9] Researchers "suggest stress [that leads to burnout] is likely the result of 'role strain,' 'role overload,' and 'spillover' from home to work and work to home," which means that burnout is not just a work problem, but is more holistic.[10]

When COVID blurred the lines between "work" and "home," it revealed just how blurred those lines have always been. In higher education, when faculty taught from home via videoconference, we had to accept that our messy home offices would be in the background, our dogs would bark, and our kids would interrupt. We had to figure out how to work in tiny spaces that were inadequate for the job. Some of us couldn't work at all because our home spaces lacked the necessary resources, and we lost our jobs. With the lines between work and home blurred, the stress between work and home blurred as well.

When faculty returned to campus, the illusion of separation did not return. Of course, for some of us, the illusion was never there in the first place. Work and home have always been blurred. This is especially true for women and other primary care providers. Pope-Ruark points out that burnout is often experienced "more deeply and regularly" by women faculty.[11] For example, there are "the challenges of the second shift, the expectations that women will do the majority of the care work for their families when they are not working." So long as women must do more at-home work, they will have that work tugging at their at-job work, and vice-versa. This push-pull existed long before the pandemic—it used to be called "work-life balance," a hilarious phrase. There is no such thing as "balance," unless you are referring to the tightrope we must walk, lest we fall into burnout. The fact is, burnout can come from any kind of labor, performed at work or at home.

But why is it that burnout, something so painful and even dangerous, can slip beneath our notice in our higher education communities? Especially after a large-scale traumatic event, when so many are experiencing it?

Systemic Burnout

Because burnout in higher education communities is so widespread, it is harder to spot. When all of our colleagues and students are suffering, suffering becomes normalized. When a problem is systemic, it becomes invisible.

I call this widespread, hard-to-spot burnout "systemic burnout." Systemic burnout is burnout caused by a large-scale traumatic event (COVID, 9/11, a school shooting) and is difficult to perceive because of its prevalence in a population. Systemic burnout is defined not only by its wide reach but also by its duration.

Systemic burnout is not the same as "institutional burnout," which happens when there is widespread burnout within an institution caused by institutional culture—like we also have in higher education. However, the two are related. For example, in addition to the systemic burnout caused by a shock event such as COVID, your college is likely also experiencing institutional burnout caused by faculty pay disparities and unreasonable work expectations. But institutional burnout is similar to systemic burnout in that they are both large scale. In fact, the institutional is often a microcosm of the societal. In this way, addressing systemic burnout at the institutional level can be an effective means, and sometimes the only means, of addressing systemic burnout.

The next time you are tempted to say, "I'm fine. After all, we are all in the same boat," stop yourself. It's true, we're all indeed in the same boat—but that boat is burning, and we are going down together unless we can spot and address systemic burnout.

Dealing with Burnout

Are you burned out? Let's revisit the symptoms that Maslach and her team point out: physical and emotional exhaustion, feelings of detachment and cynicism, and reduced feelings of efficacy and accomplishment. Basically, you are wiped out, you feel like a failure, and you believe that what you do makes no difference in the world—and furthermore, you don't care. That last part is detachment, and if you've already stopped caring, you are in the danger zone. Get help now.

Here are some red flags you can look for: missed deadlines (or more than usual), work and personal events that you keep forgetting or do not want to attend, and emails you forget or do not want to respond to. You feel overwhelmed a lot of the time. You feel like a failure a lot of the time, but you cannot explain why.

The difference between being on the edge of burnout and in the burnout zone is the difference between feeling overwhelmed but still trying and no longer trying or caring. If you are forgetting to turn something in on time, you are overwhelmed. If you are failing to turn things in on time because you cannot make yourself care, then you are burned out. If you keep forgetting to return emails, then you are overwhelmed. If you are not returning emails because you do not want to and email is stupid and pointless, then you are burned out. (I will, however, acknowledge the fact that a lot of email is, indeed, stupid and pointless.)

Large-Scale Solutions

Systemic burnout is a large-scale problem, and it requires large-scale solutions. We, as faculty and higher education institutions, cannot fix shock events like the COVID pandemic. Thus, a systemic (societal-level) solution is out of our reach. But as I noted above, the institutional is often a microcosm of the societal, as it is in the case of higher education and burnout. Thus, our higher education communities can effectively address systemic burnout at the institutional level to help faculty and students avoid burnout and recover from it.

Kevin McClure, a professor of higher education studies, points out that the burnout epidemic that arose after the pandemic was not caused by the pandemic alone, but by long-standing, exploitative higher education policies that have harmed higher education workers for decades.[12] He emphasizes that "burnout, demoralization, and disengagement aren't really about individuals waking up one day and feeling depleted or as if their professional values are being thwarted." Instead, these negative outcomes are institutional, caused by "individuals interacting with our organizations and experiencing unfair treatment, excessive workloads, chronic stress, inadequate resources, and threats to physical and social safety." What the pandemic has changed is worker outlook. That is, faculty are "less willing to blame ourselves for an inability to cope or rise above obstacles" and "our tolerance of poor working conditions has evaporated." I suggest this new intolerance is a *great* thing for faculty. It means we are demanding that institutions make changes to protect our mental health.

Institutions can use the Maslach team's causes of burnout to course correct. Thus, institutions must lighten faculty workloads, which have grown heavier and heavier over the past few decades. They must stop micromanaging their faculty and instead empower them and give them autonomy. They must repair toxic academic communities. (The next chapter addresses the toxicity in higher education.) They must fix pay and other disparities among faculty. And they must hold up their end of the bargain with their workers: if institutions expect faculty to be devoted to them, then institutions must be devoted to their faculty. If institutions want to stop faculty and students from disengaging or even fleeing their campuses, they must take a hard look at how they are treating their community members.

As McClure and Alisa Hicklin Fryar explain, faculty "disengagement" rose during COVID but only after building for years. This disengagement entails "withdrawing from certain aspects of the job or, on a more emotional level, from the institution itself," because institutions are failing to create environments in which their faculty can "flourish."[13] This faculty disengagement looks a lot like a way to protect oneself from burnout or, worse, like a consequence of burnout itself. As McClure and Fryar point out, "Research in human-resource management tells us that people need to feel safe, valued, and confident that they have the resources needed to do their jobs." They note that, for years before the pandemic, institutions already were not meeting these needs, especially for certain groups: "Women, people of color, and contingent faculty members have all had their labor exploited, and we can't argue with anyone in these groups who are re-evaluating what they are willing to give." When exploited faculty withdraw the amount of labor that they are willing to donate, institutions suffer because no one is there to pick up the slack. Institutions need to reevaluate relying on the good will of exploited faculty.

If you are looking for institutional solutions to faculty burnout, start with the faculty at the bottom of your institutional hierarchy. What extra burdens are they being asked to bear? Are they having to take care of students' mental health? (Answer: yes.) How can they be supported, institutionally? When I say "institutional support," let me be clear: I mean time, and I mean money.

Self-Care Is Not Enough

Right now, the word "self-care" as a solution for burnout is getting tossed around a lot in academia. I'm all for warm baths and meditation, but a problem arises when institutions foist the responsibility for fixing burnout onto individuals—"Just do self-care!"—without making the institutional changes necessary to relieve burnout. In this way, "do self-care" can become code for an institution passing the buck to the individual to solve a large-scale problem. I'm not saying you should not meditate or that institutions should not provide free yoga. I am saying it is not only an individual's responsibility to solve a large-scale problem.

At my institution, the University of North Carolina at Chapel Hill, the human resources website has been providing all sorts of self-care programs. There are "self-compassion" sessions (30 minutes in duration); webinars, such as "Facing Pandemic Fears with an Awake Heart" (61 minutes in duration); and more.[14] Other institutions are instituting similar programs. But when you are overworked or anxious, you do not have time—or believe that you have time—for compassion sessions, webinars, warm baths, or meditation. If you are overworked, you cannot take off two hours to go to free campus yoga. Providing free yoga without providing paid free time to do it puts the onus on the individual to make use of these campus services. That free yoga class becomes just more work. When you are already burned out or depressed, you do not have the energy to do more things.

What to Do for Yourself

If you are faculty and you are burned out, you can take steps to heal, and I strongly suggest seeking the help of a professional to do so. If you do not take steps to heal, research shows that you risk anxiety, depression, addiction, and death by suicide. Sometimes, even if you do take those steps, you will still develop a mental disability. If you are not ready or are unable to seek mental health care, there are resources you can turn to. For example, Rebecca Pope-Ruark, in her book *Unraveling Faculty Burnout*, provides a four-step process for understanding and address- ing faculty burnout that is helpful.[15]

Burnout and mental disability go hand in hand. I know that many people do not, and never will, want to identify as disabled. For many of us, identifying as disabled has been a great help, providing a community and support. But I understand the hesitation of many (if not most) fac- ulty and students to claim the identity of "mentally disabled." Academia has always been hostile to mental disability, be it temporary—like burn- out—or permanent, like bipolar disorder. Academia is where we live the "life of the mind," and your mind had better be pristine if you want to avoid stigma on the basis of your disability. By coming out as disabled, you risk your reputation, even your job. For this reason, I spent years hiding my disabilities, an exhausting task I undertook to try to pass as "normal."[16]

But even when I kept my disabilities secret from my employers, I shared it with a few trusted friends. I do recommend talking about how you feel with people you trust. I opened this chapter describing a con- versation with a friend about our mental health struggles. Friends like this one, and conversations like these, keep me going during difficult times. If you are mentally disabled, you likely have these sorts of safeties in place already. If you are experiencing mental health struggles for the first time, you need to create similar safeties for yourself—ones that feel safe to you.

4

Toxic Academic Overwork

Throughout my higher education career, I developed a terrible habit of overwork. It started as I was finishing graduate school and took my first job as a lecturer—and after that, I never held a job on the tenure track, but I never gave up hope that I would land one. No job of mine ever had a research requirement; all were teaching-only positions. Yet I never stopped publishing and presenting my research. For years, I taught up to four sections of writing, sometimes at multiple schools; then, late at night, I would stay up writing. I held out hope that if I just worked hard enough, *produced* enough, I would earn a tenure-track job.

I was wrong, of course, given higher education's addiction to contingent labor, and eventually I figured out that getting a job did not hinge on how much I published or presented at conferences. But I didn't have this epiphany until after I'd run myself ragged for nearly a decade. What kept me going all of those years? Simple: the feeling that I was a failure for never landing a tenure-track job. The thing is, many of my colleagues on the tenure track felt immense pressure as well. Sure they had landed the tenure-track job, but the fear of failing to earn tenure drove them to overwork too. There is no rest in higher ed.

Overwork is a habit that is difficult, if not impossible, to break. In academia, we must stop accepting overwork as the norm. It is toxic, and it can be deadly—many of us have learned firsthand how overwork can lead to mental health struggles, including burnout, anxiety, depression, and more.

The Toxic Source

Toxic overwork in higher education has its roots in institutional—not individual—belief systems. Over the past fifty years, higher education has become more and more market-driven. It relies more on contingent faculty labor, taking money from secure faculty jobs and pushing it toward glossy new campus facilities.[1] Despite the shrinking number of faculty jobs, the demand for faculty output has only risen. Research shows how institutional toxicity harms faculty. One negative outcome of "the drive for increased performance" by faculty is "a hyper-competitive and individualistic working environment."[2] In this competitive environment, faculty have stopped caring about collegial relationships because they are "addicted to optimization and efficiency."[3] This individualistic environment creates a culture where one colleague's failure works to another's benefit, and there is no incentive to help one another succeed. Furthermore, perceived weakness is not tolerated. As professor and burnout expert Rebecca Pope-Ruark explains, "Being weak or making work for others because you can't handle [the impossible expectations of higher education]—these are things you just don't do if you want to develop or maintain your credibility as a serious academic."[4]

Pope-Ruark describes her own experience with academic overwork and how it is linked to a fear of failure: "Higher-ed culture told me that my worth was based on my productivity; that I was only as good as the number of articles I published, the scores I received on my end-of-semester student evaluations, the level at which I could compete with other scholars to increase the reputation of my institution, and the sheer number of hours I dedicated to 'doing' higher ed."[5] As Pope-Ruark describes, academia's culture of toxic overwork made her believe that her value as a person was tied to her production. If she stopped producing, she would be a failure. But Pope-Ruark's overwork eventually led to terrible career burnout and depression.

Individual higher education workers are not going to dismantle the market-driven machine that higher education has become anytime soon (but the upswing in labor organizing over the past decade is inspiring). However, we can protect ourselves from the pressures it exerts as best we can. We can, collectively and individually, open our eyes to the institutional pressure to overwork and resist it. We can recognize that overwork is not a norm we must live with but an abusive demand that we deserve to protect ourselves from.

Reframing Failure

Toxic overwork sneaks up on academics because it tells us a lie: it promises that it will prevent failure. To a group conditioned to crave perfection, the lie is enticing. As neuroscience professor Hilal A. Lashuel explains, our academic peers rarely view failure as the learning experience that it is, but as a sign that "we are not fit for academia." Because failure is anathema in higher education, he writes, it is "not the place where we are likely to get second chances." [6] Our fear of failure drives us to overwork as a way of protecting ourselves from the black mark failure would leave on our careers. Overwork gives us a false sense of control, leading us to believe that failure can be avoided or buried under a mountain of successes. (It can't.)

If we can let go of the fear of failure, we are one step closer to breaking the bad habit of overwork. Law professor and academic success professional Kaci Bishop is an expert on failure in higher education. She observes that, among professors and students alike, "Failure is treated like the other F word. It suggests finality and is stigmatizing and associated with guilt, blame, and shame. Something people understandably want to ignore or sweep under the rug."[7] She points out the type of person who is most vulnerable to the negative outcomes of failure—perfectionists: "Unsurprisingly, individuals who tend to be perfectionists or who have perfectionistic tendencies set 'exceedingly high standards of performance' and are thus more apt to be negatively impacted or 'overly self-critical' when that performance falls short of expectations." Perfectionism is one of the most toxic driving forces behind academia, leading faculty to believe that if one's work isn't perfect, it is therefore a failure.

Perfectionism also gets in the way of successfully managing *actual* failures. Bishop notes that perfectionism can become destructive over time, particularly in environments, such as higher education, where the focus is on outcomes and production. Perfectionism destroys a person's ability to take feedback and to hear criticism because they are less willing to admit they've made mistakes. Mistakes, after all, are failures, and failures are unacceptable. But if a person does not address their failures and learn from them, they can get stuck in what Bishop calls a "perfection-paralysis cycle," unable to move past their failures or learn from them, making the same mistakes over and over. One of those mistakes that many of us make is overwork.

Overwork and Anxiety

Like many faculty, I have coped with fear of failure by overworking, which in turn led to immense stress and anxiety. At the same time, my fear of failure is caused by perfectionism, which in turn is a symptom of my anxiety disorder. In short, overwork and anxiety are inextricably linked. Many faculty, even those without anxiety disorders, face a cycle of overwork: the fear of failure leads to overwork, which creates stress and anxiety. The anxiety in turn leads back to fear of failure, and the cycle starts again.

Many faculty in higher education have anxiety disorders; a 2018 study found anxiety disorders among 39 percent of faculty and staff.[8] It seems that the prevalence of anxiety disorders creates the urge for perfectionism and the fear of failure. It also seems that a high-pressure environment that demands perfectionism can cause immense stress and anxiety. I suggest there is no point in trying to parse whether the pressure for perfection in academia leads to anxiety or whether anxiety creates the need for perfection. We must simply face the problem at hand: high rates of anxiety and overwork.

Generally, if you have an anxiety disorder, you believe you can protect yourself against things that go wrong if you just do (or do not do) other things. (I discuss anxiety in more detail in Chapter 1.) In the context of overwork, you might react to perceived uncertainty with overwork, hoping the overwork will soothe the uncertainty. And the process works—for a little while. The uncertainty is soothed for an hour, or a day. But then the uncertainty returns, so you overwork again. The uncertainty, the *fear*, pushes you furiously. You believe you can protect yourself against failure if you just do more, and more, and then even more.

When we run ourselves into the ground with overwork, we can damage our health. As Lashuel explains, "Often, we do not realize until it is too late that poor work-life balance and pretending that we are on top of everything"—typical academic behavior—"comes at a great cost to our health, wellbeing and our families."[9] Toxic academic overwork can lead to mental and physical health issues: "Pressure, stress and anxiety frequently translate into sleep deprivation, exhaustion, irritability and isolation, all of which negatively affects our quality of life and our inter-actions with students and colleagues." The toxicity cycle affects not just the person dealing with it, but everyone around them.

This toxicity can have very real ramifications for faculty. Lashuel writes, "Chronic stress [from academic culture] is also a major risk fac-tor for developing many psychiatric and cardiovascular disorders."[10] Lashuel himself had a near-deadly awakening that led him to write about mental health and higher education: he suffered two heart at-tacks in three years. Lashuel's heart attacks led him to reframe his en-tire academic working life for the better. He recognized the fears and toxicity that surrounded him, he set better boundaries, and he even be-came "more sensitive to the struggles of those around [him]" and now encourages them to "share their mental health challenges" with him, providing support to others.

But, as I have explained throughout this book, being open about one's mental health struggles is not an option for many in higher education because it puts their jobs at risk. As disability studies scholar Margaret Price points out, disclosing a mental disability such as an anxiety disor-der in higher education can be dangerous. The stigma against mental disability plays out in the "popular conception that unsound minds have no place in the classroom."[11] For faculty, she points out, the consequence of this belief is that perceived "'unstable' or 'difficult' teachers" lose their jobs. Pope-Ruark felt such fear once she was diagnosed with burnout: "I completely believed that admitting I was well and truly burned out would be disastrous to my career."[12] The need for secrecy about men-tal disability and mental health struggles, driven by the stigma against mental disability, prevents intervention in the toxicity cycle. So long as there is a stigma against mental disability in academia, anyone strug-gling with their mental health will be afraid to seek help.

Overwork Starts Early

Academics are trained to overwork early, starting in graduate school, when we learn quickly to say yes to every opportunity that comes our way: every panel, every book review, every anything that might push our job application up a little higher in the desperate queue for a job. The academic job market has been tough for a long time now, to the point that to say no to anything as a graduate student feels like a career-ending move.

We must take a look at how we teach our graduate students—even our undergraduates. What are we teaching them about what it means to be successful? Do we require them to overwork? Probably. Instead, can we teach them to set boundaries? Can we teach them the life skill of asking for deadline extensions so that they can do so fearlessly and avoid turning in late or shoddy work? As we face our own challenges in the workplace, we can simultaneously improve the lives of our students.

Unfortunately, these bad overwork habits do not stay isolated in our work lives—they spill over into everything we do. Because of overwork, I missed my son's first steps; I was attending my fourth academic conference of the year. As I was sitting at a table in the hotel bar, my spouse called me joyously and sent me a video. After we hung up, I cried. You cannot leave your bad overwork habits at work. You bring them home with you; you cannot help it. Because overwork is a habit, it must be broken everywhere.

Institutions Must Combat Toxicity

Toxicity and overwork in higher education are not problems that individuals can fix. They are "organizational problems that require organizational solutions,"[13] as Kevin McClure, a professor of higher education studies, puts it. McClure has studied the "Great Resignation" post-COVID pandemic and notes that, although the pandemic provided the "spark" for the nationwide worker disengagement, burnout, and departure from higher education, the "fuel" for it has been amassing for decades. That is, working conditions on campus have grown worse and worse over the years long before the pandemic forced many of us to reckon with them.[14] These poor working conditions arose from long-standing policies that have led to "unfair treatment at work," "unreasonable time pressures," "leaders who aren't listening, low compensation, and understaffing" and more. The culture of overwork in higher education has not arisen in a vacuum; it is institutionally supported. If you are underpaid, and doing extra work will earn you the few more bucks you need to make ends meet, you will do that work. In higher education, toxic overwork is a feature, not a bug.

This feature has created a culture where overwork is praised among faculty and even bragged about. Pope-Ruark describes "the cult of busyness that has cursed so many of us to fetishize productivity and reputation."[15] This busyness problem is institutional, rooted in "the systematic structures" of academia itself. Thus, many faculty do not seek help for the stress and anxiety that drive them to overwork, because they believe that overwork is normal and to fail at overwork is to fail at academia.

Later, when these struggles become a crisis, they do not seek help because mental health struggles are taboo in academia. So they keep them secret and face declining mental health. If institutions want to support faculty (and students) in seeking help for mental health struggles, they must start at the root: the stigma against mental disabilities. Stigma creates negative stereotyping and isolation of mentally disabled people, typically based on irrational fear of undesirable behavior such as irresponsibility, instability, or violence. Stigma also works internally on disabled people themselves, creating feelings of isolation and shame.

To eradicate stigma, institutions must adopt inclusive practices, which require taking active steps to welcome mentally disabled people into academia, a community that has previously shamed and excluded them. In such an inclusive community, all community members will feel safe discussing mental health—and toxicity will have a much harder time taking root.

If institutions were to support faculty mental health, they would be taking a step in helping break the toxicity cycle of academia that we have taken for granted for far too long. Doing so will create a healthier workplace with less turnover, greater faculty engagement, better communication between all members of an institution, and better teaching and role-modeling for students.

The new market-driven university may be here to stay, but we can improve the conditions under which we work. We can hold our institutions accountable by protecting our mental health, fighting institutional stigma against mental disabilities, and setting boundaries in the workplace to nurture a healthy career.

5

Setting Boundaries

When I was a young professor, I had a wonderful mentor. One day, I approached her with a conundrum. I'd received an invitation to give a talk (unpaid) at a conference on the other side of the country—I live in North Carolina, and the conference was in Seattle.

"I feel like I have to say yes," I said. "It's such a wonderful invitation."

"It *is* a wonderful invitation," she said. "But you don't have to say yes."

A few years prior to this conversation, I would have said yes without hesitation. After all, I was a non-tenure-track professor constantly trying to prove my worth to my colleagues—plus I have anxiety disorder, which means I am constantly worried about my self-worth. The toxic culture of academic overwork had me in its jaws.

But that day, I hesitated because I'd had a baby a few months earlier, and I also had a two-year-old at home. And since this speaking engagement would be my fifth that year, the parental guilt, and exhaustion, were kicking in.

Nevertheless, I was wrestling with the decision of whether to accept an unpaid invited talk, my fifth in one year, at a conference that would require two days for the travel alone, while having a newborn and a toddler at home, for a job that did not require such work, with the hope that I would somehow prove myself to be a "real" professor to my colleagues, a laughable goal. In retrospect, the decision seems like an easy "no." But it was not easy at the time.

"How can I possibly say no?" I said to my mentor.

"It's simple. You say, 'I'm honored to be invited, but I must decline.'"

I recall laughing at her words, which did seem so simple, even as the knot of anxiety in my belly wound tighter at the thought of writing them in an email.

"I can't," I said.

She paused. "Why are you afraid to say no?" she finally asked. Then she put her finger right on the sore spot. "Are you afraid they'll never ask you again?" I knew that the "they" in her sentence encompassed far more than the conference organizers. The "they" referred to anyone who might ever invite me to do something important again. And she was right. I told them no and did not regret it.

Stepping back, I could see that I was afraid to set a boundary. Anne Katherine, expert on interpersonal boundaries, describes them this way: "Boundaries define what is you and what is not you, what matters to you, and what doesn't matter. They are a container for positive actions and choices, and restrict intrusions, distractions, and detours."[1] For me, saying no to the Seattle conference entailed setting a positive personal boundary. The boundary prioritized my mental health, personal time, and young family. But boundary-setting in higher education isn't easy. You aren't setting boundaries against mere people, but against immense institutional pressures that encourage faculty to overwork, endlessly prove themselves, and constantly create academic "product." If you are marginalized faculty, boundary-setting is even harder because we are expected to take on even more than our fair share of labor. And, if you are one of the many faculty who have anxiety disorders (see Chapter 1), setting a boundary can be terrifying.

Do not despair if you at first find it hard to set boundaries. Katherine writes, "Boundary setting is a skill, like reading, skating, or watering plants. The first time you do it, it feels awkward and unnatural." But the more you set boundaries, the easier it becomes to do so. The first few times, however, can be really, really hard.

Boundaries and Vulnerable Faculty

In higher education (and elsewhere), fear of negative consequences often drives the fear of setting boundaries. This fear is especially powerful for "vulnerable faculty," as law professor Meera Deo describes them: a group that includes "women of color, caregivers, white women, and untenured."[2] Vulnerable faculty also includes all faculty of color, graduate students, and, of course, disabled faculty. Our fear of setting boundaries did not arise from nowhere. If you are vulnerable in academia and try to set a boundary, there may very well be negative consequences. Those with power in academia are not accustomed to hearing the word "no," especially from those whom they are most comfortable bossing around.

But, for me, a mentally disabled woman and primary caregiver working off the tenure track, these real risks led me to believe that I had to say yes to everything. I could not discern the difference between saying yes to appease a departmental bully, which felt like a necessary evil, and safely turning down an opportunity that I did not have time for.

Deo also points out that the fear of future rejection due to boundary-setting haunts certain faculty more than it does others. Women of color, white women, and caregivers struggle with this fear the most, leading them to say yes too frequently and for too little reward.

Throughout academia, there are expectations that marginalized faculty must do more than their colleagues. For example, a plethora of research shows that women faculty members do significantly more service work than their male colleagues.[3] At the same time, the academy holds women to higher standards in teaching and scholarship when it comes time for hiring and review. The double bind is that the service work women are expected to perform cuts into the time that women have to do scholarship. Gender also intersects with the types of faculty positions women hold. As professors Renee Allen, Alicia Jackson, and DeShun Harris have pointed out, women hold a disproportionate number of contingent faculty positions.[4] The authors term this contract work with heavy workloads and low pay the "pink ghetto." If you work in a contract position as a primary caregiver and identify as a woman, you likely feel more insecure than other faculty when trying to set boundaries.

Black faculty and other faculty of color bear an enormous burden in higher education. In the foundational study "Maids of Academe: African American Women Faculty at Predominately White Institutions," Debra A. Harley documents "the disproportionate role African American women assume in service, teaching, and research" at predominantly white colleges and universities (i.e., ones that are not Historically Black Colleges and Universities [HBCUs]).[5] Latino scholar Amado M. Padilla writes about the "cultural taxation"[6] that ethnic minorities must pay when the administration of a predominantly white institution "assumes that we are best suited for specific tasks because of our race/ethnicity or our presumed knowledge of cultural differences."[7] This labor, Padilla explains, is "very time consuming and often emotionally draining," and it gives little professional reward because "service on behalf of cultural diversity is not usually in the equation for promotion within academia."[8] Scholars have pointed out how Black, Indigenous, and people of color (BIPOC) faculty (as well as students) "are commonly burdened with the task of identifying and raising DEIA [diversity, equity, inclusion, and antiracism] issues to the attention" of school administrations.[9] The problem is that "being the community member that always raises issues comes at political costs, particularly for nontenured faculty, who may be branded by administrators or colleagues as someone who is 'difficult,' impolite, and even, at times, too revolutionary."[10] Thus, although the institutional burden of this work falls to BIPOC faculty, at the same time, BIPOC faculty doing this work may be risking their careers—yet another double bind. Do you set a boundary and say no to this work, risking your career? Or do you do this work and risk your career?

Disability Accommodations: Trampling Boundaries

The vast majority of mentally disabled faculty (and students) do not seek campus accommodations for their disabilities.[11] One reason is that the process is so invasive. As a disabled person seeking accommodations in higher education, you are not permitted to have personal boundaries. This trampling of privacy is one of the many flaws of the accommodations model and how it is used in the United States today.

A disabled faculty member cannot enter the human resources department of their institution or department, state that they are disabled, describe the accommodations they need, and receive them. Instead, they must submit to an invasive examination and verification of their disability.[12] The issue is one of mistrust of disabled people. Institutions do not trust disabled people to serve as witnesses to their own disabilities and needs; they also do not trust that disabled people aren't faking. Thus, institutions require medical evidence to prove that a disabled person is truly disabled. In our society, we take it for granted that this proof is required by law, even though it is not—the law permits it but does not require it.

Thus, if you are a faculty member seeking accommodations, you must provide extensive documentation about your disability, including wide access to your medical records. Once you hand these records over to your institution, they are stored in a campus office that is far less secure than a medical practice. As one disabled faculty member described the process, "The documentation I was required to provide once I disclosed my disability made me feel that I was being forced to put my various symptoms on display for public consumption."[13] This same faculty member believed that "this hurdle will surely cause other academics to avoid disclosure" of their disabilities.

Another reason mentally disabled people do not disclose their disabilities on campus, of course, is stigma and the fear of negative repercussions. Thus, sometimes the only way to maintain personal boundaries between oneself and the institution with regard to one's mental disability is by not seeking accommodations and by keeping the disability secret.

And here, again, we find a double bind. You can either disclose your disability for needed accommodations and risk invasion of privacy and negative community repercussions. Or you can choose not to disclose your disability and suffer the negative repercussions that come from the hard work of hiding your disability.

Some Boundaries We Can Set

Despite all of these risks, it is important for our mental health to learn to set boundaries. You must assess the risks that you are willing to take. For my part, I discovered that saying no in some circumstances was less risky than I had imagined it to be. I hope the same is true for you. Here are some ideas for how to set boundaries.

Reevaluate deadlines. Do you feel bound by deadlines, afraid of the negative consequences of breaking them? Have you ever worked through a weekend or late nights to meet an impossible deadline, hating yourself the whole time? (I have.) As law professor Sarah J. Schendel points out, many faculty end up "swamped by tasks," because they are "imperfect at prioritization, and either confused or aggravated by the work of anticipating deadlines and asking for extensions."[14] The point is, you are not alone. Asking for reasonable deadlines, and for extensions when you need them, is one way to set good boundaries.

In the context of vulnerable faculty, however, some of us feel that asking for extensions is not an option for us. Vulnerable faculty feel less empowered to ask for extensions because we believe it reflects badly on our work, and sometimes—to some of our colleagues—it does. They believe we should be at their beck and call. Because of these pressures, we do not believe that extensions are even an option for us. But they are. We can push back slowly, train these colleagues who trample our boundaries that their behavior is unacceptable. Doing so can be terrifying at first, but we must protect ourselves or we will break down.

Here's a helpful script for asking for an extension: "I find I am unable to complete the project by the deadline. I will need another two weeks. Thank you for your understanding." Notice that there are no excuses or explanations. Notice also that there is a thank you at the end of that script, but there is no endless stream of apologies. Why? You have nothing to apologize for. You are merely stating facts. You will get the work done. You need two more weeks. Of course, if you are missing a deadline with big ramifications for other people (and you would be surprised how few of these there are), you can do more than provide notification. You can suggest a way to meet the deadline, say, by suggesting a replacement for you. But the fact remains, it is better to set the boundary than fail to meet an unmeetable deadline—even if you did not know it would be unmeetable when you took on the project. After all, you could not predict when your dog would need surgery or your kid's daycare would close because of a norovirus. Life happens.

You also do not need to jump to reply to emails right away. Author Melissa Febos takes on this issue in her funny yet sharp essay on the inequities that exist in replying to emails ("Do You Want to Be Known for Your Writing, or For Your Swift Email Responses?"). "We [women-identifying people] are conditioned to ever prove ourselves, as if our value is contingent on our ability to meet the expectations of others." Febos continues: "Our worth is a tank forever draining that we must fill and fill. We complete tasks and in some half-buried way believe that if we don't, we will be discredited."[15] One way we fill this tank is to jump to reply to emails as fast as possible. And when we don't reply immediately, we apologize profusely for taking so long to do so. Vulnerable faculty feel a constant need to prove that we are valuable members of a faculty. And it is true that our institutions frequently hold us to higher standards. But Febos provides (albeit wry and sometimes cynical) advice for how to lower others' expectations of us. Simply this: stop replying to emails so quickly. Let them sit a day. But the bigger picture of her essay is this: we have trained others to count on us to do too much.

Setting boundaries will enable us to push back against unreasonable expectations that cause us to run ourselves into the ground. But fighting the overwork that vulnerable faculty face is not only an individual task, it is institutional. The boundaries that we must put up, even if they seem to be between ourselves and colleagues, are actually between us and unreasonable and inequitable institutional expectations. These institutional expectations of vulnerable faculty insist that we perform more service duties than other, less vulnerable faculty. Therefore, to reject those service duties can have negative professional consequences. Figuring out which things to say no to can be like walking a tightrope.

What we can do is this: recognize that while some of these expectations come from external sources, many come from within ourselves, from our own internalized beliefs about what we should do. Setting boundaries as a white woman, a disabled woman, a woman of color, or any other vulnerable faculty member has risks, but we can learn to accurately identify and navigate them. Not only can we, but we must—in order to preserve our mental health and, hopefully, create organized change from inside an institutional structure that demands we do too much.

6

The Disabled Mind in Academia

Outside of the conference hotel, I could not see a body. What I did see, as my cab pulled into the circular drive, were multiple police cars with their lights strobing, yellow tape blocking most of the road, a large black van, and crime scene investigators, including one with an oversized camera and a flash the size of a dinner plate.

These are objects that any lawyer or other person trained like me knows accompany the dead.

As he checked me in, the concierge said, "There's been an accident. I'm sorry if traffic was jammed."

Traffic had indeed been jammed. When I saw the scene, I knew why.

I resisted the urge to ask him if he knew details about the scene. Instead I thanked him and took my room key and headed to a tall tower overlooking Tampa Bay.

It was 2015, and I was in Tampa to participate in a scholarly conference. The next day, I would present on a disability studies panel about mental illness. Although I had recently left my full-time teaching job, I still wanted to come and give this talk. My previous job was as a contingent faculty member, where I was paid only to teach, not to do research. But I did do research, in particular in disability studies. I had smart colleagues around the country, and this panel was a capstone of a recent project that I had proposed with two of them before I left my job.

After entering my room and dropping my bag on the floor, I rushed to the window for an overhead view of the scene. I was compelled by a need I did not understand. The scene was on a small bridge connecting two spits of land, each spit covered in hotels and tourist-centric restaurants. Through my window, I could make out only the white tail of one of the police cruisers.

Moments later, the same compulsion led me to the elevators, through the lobby, and back outside. At the time, if you had asked me why I was going to the scene, I would have told you that I possessed the same grim fascination as anyone else when confronted by a tragic accident. But that answer would not have been the truth. I was not a typical onlooker.

When I reached the bridge, I didn't rubberneck. I dissected. I already knew that the accident was unusual based on the details I'd seen from the cab; I learned even more from the details I gathered from outside the police tape.

And I was riveted.

As I took in those details, my ears filled with an internal whoosh that blocked out the sounds around me. I was barely aware of the other conference-goers who passed by me on the unblocked portion of the bridge, heading to lunches and gatherings, doing what I should have been doing. But I couldn't understand how they could go about their day when a massive tragedy had transpired only inches from them only minutes before. But even then I knew: I was the one who was off-kilter, not them.

Yellow plastic numbers pockmarked the bridge. On her knees, the crime scene photographer took a photo by number three. I knelt as well, noticing that number three marked a bloodstain on the pale pavement. Now dried, the bloodstain looked like a streak of brown paint. Over by number five lay a damp navy-blue strip of fabric.

The camera's flash burst brightly even in the Florida daylight. I followed each burst, tracking each piece of evidence. Step by meticulous step, these workers reconstructed a killing.

The conference happened a decade ago. At the time, it was plain to me that a death had occurred, but I had not felt horror—I had felt fascination. I had also felt dissociated from my own body, which I had left behind to enter a bubble. Inside of that bubble was just me and the scene, and the background noises, people, even buildings fell away. I wanted to get closer, even closer. At the time, I could not have told you why. I could not have said that my brain was twirling a question: *What if that had been me?*

It took me a while to unpack my feelings about that day. I felt fixated, but I did not feel ghoulish. I knew I was not gawking, but I could not explain how what I was doing was not gawking. What I did not realize at the time was this: I could see the empty space where the body had been, and in that empty space I saw my own dead body.

At that disability conference, where I was going to talk about mental disability, my own brush with suicide was thrust before me as I arrived in my taxi. But at the time, my mental disability was still a secret I kept close except from a select few, fearing backlash from colleagues, superiors, and even students at my former institution, where my contingent professor job was insecure. I even feared backlash from my fellow conference-goers, who would have viewed a person with bipolar disorder with fear and disgust—as research shows that most people in the United States do.[1]

Critical Distance

Later, once the details of the accident hit the news, I learned the rest of what happened on the bridge. In a crowded, tourist-filled area of Tampa, a driver lost control of a car at high speed and tore through pedestrian traffic. The car struck and killed a person, who died at the scene. From what I pieced together, the coroner and crime scene technicians took the body away approximately thirty minutes before my arrival.

In the hours before the news of the death publicly broke, I felt like I held a secret, one I couldn't share. I didn't know how to explain to my colleagues about the scene. What would I have said without sounding strange? Who was so fascinated with death at a place where people come together to celebrate friendship? I tried to imagine how this conversation would go, and every time it went poorly:

> Me: Someone died out on that bridge. The police are treating it as a homicide.
> *An awkward silence.*
> Them: Um, okay. How can you tell?
> Me: There are numbers, and some blood. And the techs don't document a scene like that unless it's—well, it's hard to explain. It's the gestalt of the thing.
> Them: A gestalt told you the accident was what, a *murder*?

In my mind, the person's discomfort would be palpable, and I would have caused it.

Of course, it is possible that I was wrong about how my colleagues would have reacted to my story about the scene. But at the time, I was too intimidated to try. The secret felt vulnerable.

The secret wasn't even that there was a death on the bridge. No, my secret was, *This particular kind of death is close to me.* The other part of the secret was this: I have bipolar disorder, and I have come close to suicide.

I couldn't reveal my feelings about the body without revealing why I had them.

By that evening, the first night of the conference, all everyone was talking about was the person who died. In the packed lobby of the conference hotel, the story passed from person to person, from table to table, and my secret was no longer a secret.

That night, I went to dinner with one of my co-panelists, a good friend and disability studies professor named Kat. I told her about arriving and going straight out to the scene, how I could not look away from it.

I said, "I can't figure out why I'm so emotional about it. It's not like I've never seen a crime scene before."

She grabbed my hand. "Jesus, Katie. It must have been so hard for you."

"It was," I said, but I was baffled by her intensity, which seemed more than the situation warranted. I paused, nonplussed. "What are you saying?"

And then, with her words, the memory came back: how, just a few months before, in the middle of the night, I walked onto a dark road, hoping to die. I snuck out of my house, dressed in black, and walked the unlit streets of our miserable neighborhood, daring a car to come along and strike me down. No one did. So I returned home, quietly entered my house again, and told no one for months. Not my therapist, not my spouse.

A useful term for my actions is "parasuicide," which is "any nonfatal, self-injurious behavior with a clear intent to cause bodily harm or death."[2] That night, I put myself in harm's way on purpose, knowing I could be struck and killed at any time. I played a dangerous game of chance. Kat was one of the very few people who knew my secret. As soon as she said those words—*It must have been so hard for you*—I knew that she was right.

Earlier that day, when I had seen death in the crime scene details, I had seen myself. Without realizing it at the time, I had stood at the side of the road that afternoon to mourn. I mourned for myself, upset that I had ever reached a place so low, and for my family, whose health and happiness I put in danger when I put myself in danger. I didn't know the person who had died on the bridge. I didn't know if they were a man or a woman. I only knew that it could have been me—differently than the way my conference peers may also have thought, *It could have been me*.

No really. It could have been me. At another time, on another street.

Once you have brushed up against suicide, death becomes your neighbor always. You become accustomed to it, attuned.

On the bridge, part of me thought, I am a person with bipolar disorder who once sank so deep in depression that I contemplated walking into a dark street to die.

That contemplation, and the dark walk that followed it, had happened not long before, but I had forgotten about it entirely, in the way psychology research shows that a person forgets what happens when they are depressed.[3] I think it's the brain's way of saving you from the worst times of your life, like the amnesia people feel after giving birth. If we could remember the pain, we would never have another child. The amnesia is a survival device.

If I could remember the pain of depression, I certainly would not have gone to a conference to present on mental disability. No, I would have eaten microwave nachos and slept on my couch, hair dirty and mind adrift. How could there be a point to anything if it could all go to shit so quickly and for no reason?

I would never have been able to talk publicly and with critical distance about a thing if it had continued to sit so heavily on my shoulders. But it did not.

Epistemic Injustice

Before I left full-time higher education, I regularly attended this conference, which I particularly enjoyed because of its strong disability studies presence. Disability studies was my niche. I wrote scholarship and gave talks about how mentally disabled people are demonized in the media, ostracized by society, and scapegoated by politicians and our judicial system. For example, in a study of public perceptions of mental illness, 33 percent of study participants reported that they believed people with major depressive disorder were likely to be violent toward others.[4] (They are not.)

Back then, I stood up in front of rooms filled with people, and I spoke sensible, rational words, arguing, in academic terms, for greater rights for mentally disabled people. I did so because, as disability studies pioneer Lennard Davis writes, disability studies functions "both as an academic discipline and as an area of political struggle."[5] But back then I would never have revealed that I, too, am a person who is demonized, ostracized, and scapegoated. That I, too, have a mental disability (bipolar disorder) that most people in the United States find terrifying—including other disabled people.

Of course, when I'm depressed, I cannot muster up the energy to feel violent toward anything, except maybe the remote control if it isn't working properly. There is an enormous gap between the public perception and the reality of what it means to be depressed, to have anxiety disorder, to be autistic, and so on.

As a disability studies expert, I am very familiar with the research on that gap. I am also familiar with the pain that mentally disabled people often feel when their identity—their entire being—is subsumed by their disability. Psychology researchers describe an "epistemic injustice" that happens "when the subordinate party [the mentally disabled person] is not regarded as a credible or reliable knower by the dominant party"—say, the judicial system, or school system or, basically, all of society—"for reasons that are irrelevant to the subordinate party's capacities as a knower."[6] In other words, this type of injustice occurs when a mentally disabled person's very ability to make decisions, observe their world, or witness their own pain is tied only to their identity as mentally disabled—which is irrelevant to their ability to do those things. (Yes, it is.) Why? Because the "dominant party" makes decisions that "depend rather on negative stereotypes associated with the subordinate party's identity" instead of their actual ability to make decisions or know things. For example, a patient might go to the doctor with chronic headaches, and the doctor might say, "These are caused by your anxiety," rather than doing a full workup such as looking into concussion history or family history of migraines. Even when the patient insists that their anxiety has nothing to do with the headaches, the doctor will not listen because the patient is not "a credible or reliable knower." (I'm describing a precise experience that happened to me.)

My colleagues in rhetoric studies would call my experience with the doctor and the headaches a "loss of rhetoricity," that is, an inability to participate in public discourse, which happens because mentally disabled people are deemed unreliable. As disability studies scholar Catherine Prendergast has famously written, "To be disabled mentally is to be disabled rhetorically."[7] My doctor found my description of my symptoms unreliable because of my disability. Indeed, I approach every interaction with every medical provider with caution, knowing that at the top of my medical record are two diagnoses that tank my credibility in the eyes of many medical professionals: bipolar disorder and anxiety disorder. To many doctors, every word I speak is suspect.

Compulsory Disclosure

Yet, despite the many negative outcomes that accompany disclosure of mental disability, there are some scholars in disability studies who argue for compulsory disclosure of disabled status. Disability studies (DS) scholar Corbett J. O'Toole expressed frustration that scholars do not disclose their disabled status in a 2013 article ("Disclosing Our Relationships to Disabilities: An Invitation for Disability Studies Scholars").[8] She advocates for posing this question at every panel at DS conferences: "What is your relationship to disability?" Her argument for "universal public disclosure" of disability status at DS conferences is that it will "challenge the shame typically associated with identifying with disabled people." In her view, if all DS scholars disclose, they will "symbolically demonstrate the positive value of the disabled experience." She also argues that disclosure will move a disabled person "from isolation to community." Although O'Toole suggests disability status must be shared, she allows that disabled people can keep their "medical information" such as diagnoses "private" because some disabilities (like, say, mine) are highly stigmatized.

My marginalia on O'Toole's article are not fit for public consumption. It mostly boils down to this: never once in her article does she mention contingent employment or job security. She mentions that "publicly naming our relationship to disability is not always easy or comfortable," but she is wrong—for many of us, it is dangerous. At one point she asks, "Why the fear and trepidation about public knowledge" about disability status? But she does not push her inquiry to find an answer. She does not ask a person who is actually afraid.

I can answer that question—I have answered it publicly, many times. When I was a full-time contingent faculty member with a hidden disability, I was afraid I would lose my job if someone found out about it. I am still afraid I will get poor medical care. I am afraid neighbors will not let their children come over to play at my house with my kids—they will not say why, it will just . . . happen. Newscasters speculate whether spree killers have my diagnoses. Already I cannot get life insurance. I barely pass the test for TSA PreCheck. The rights and privileges of a person who lives in the United States are severely limited when you have my disabilities.

Despite all of these dangers, once I was no longer at risk of being fired and losing my health insurance, I did disclose. I chose the activist route. But I did it for all of the others who could not. I have immense respect for those who decide to keep their disabilities secret, out of the public eye, or within their private disability communities, because I know how dangerous it is to disclose on any public platform. Even if the disclosure is simply "I am disabled," a person is taking a risk. If O'Toole thinks that everyone in the audience will resist speculating just *how* a person is disabled, she is naive. If she thinks a DS conference is somehow free of ableism and stigma, she is worse than naive.

Demanding disabled people who are early-career, graduate students, or contingent to disclose anything about their disabilities is wildly unfair. Faculty with insecure employment face even more challenges when disclosing than those with tenure and therefore greater job security. Kate Kaul ("Risking Experience") writes about the intersection of contingent academic jobs and the disclosure of disabilities, pointing out how either of those factors—insecure employment or mental disability—can put an academic career in jeopardy.[9]

First, simply being contingent faculty can get you stuck in a contingent career forever because you become "stale" in a job market that only wants fresh new faces out of their doctoral programs. Kaul writes that "even representing oneself as an adjunct [i.e., as contingent] can be disastrous for an academic career."[10] Many others have pointed out the same. As Kelly J. Baker et al. note, empirical research shows that "the farther a PhD is from their degree, the less hirable they seem."[11]

Job insecurity and disability are a dangerous mix. Sometimes an academic chooses to disclose for beneficial professional reasons, but with that disclosure come professional risks. For a contingent faculty member those risks can be profound. As Kaul writes, "For disabled academics, disclosure is sometimes a claim to authority and experience."[12] For me, as a disability studies scholar and expert, acknowledging my disability gives me the authority of lived experience, it is true. But, Kaul notes, "in my own experience [Kaul is a contingent faculty member]—a claim to authority is a small compensation for the risks that disclosure exposes me to when I ask for accommodation."

For example, when you have a contingent position, teaching is frequently your only job. As Kaul points out, disclosing a disability can have a potential negative influence on your course evaluations.[13] Course evaluations are the top metric that determine the retention of contingent faculty. If your evaluations are poor, you might not have your contract renewed. In this way, being a contingent faculty and disclosing your disability can harm your career. Stigma follows disability all over the ivory tower: from the faculty lounge and into the classroom. Only those who have bulletproof careers can truly risk that stigma without fear of repercussions.

Pressured to Disclose

The year before, at this same conference, in 2014, I presented on the stigma against mental illness, the gun control debate, and how news coverage of spree killing excludes the voices of mentally disabled journalists. After all, in our ableist society, disclosure of mental disability would hurt a journalist's credibility as an impartial writer on the topic.

After my panelists and I delivered our talks, during the question-and-answer session, a young disability studies scholar stood up. With their dark hair, dark eyes, and intense stare, they said, "Do any of you identify as disabled?" The question was startling, and my heart started racing. That risk to credibility I spoke about? I wasn't speaking hypothetically or theoretically. I was speaking about myself.

After the audience member asked the question, my co-panelists each answered in the negative.

Then it was my turn. I was shaking with fear. I wanted to run from the room or scream at the young person who had asked the question. I was terrified and furious at the same time.

I spoke calmly, though. "I have a psychiatric disability," I said.

At the time, I was still employed as a contingent faculty member. I never spoke about my disability in public. But I couldn't lie—I'm terrible at it. And it isn't how I'm wired. Perhaps it is because I'm autistic; perhaps it is something else. For whatever reason, I told the truth.

The person's question was a test, and I did not like it. I wanted to rage at the danger they had put me in—real danger, even if they could not see it.

I wish, now, that I had pushed back against the question instead of freezing like a rabbit. I wish I had said something about my job security: "You are putting my job at risk by asking this question." I wish I had given my opinion about forced outing: "I don't agree with being asked this question in a public forum. It is not the duty of disabled scholars to put themselves at risk of scapegoating and stigma for the greater good of disability studies as a field."

But I did not. So I am doing it now.

Disclosure Blues

At the Tampa conference, I responded directly to my experience the year before. By then I was out of academia, and I told the story of the forced outing and how it affected me.

I said, Disclosure of mental disabilities in higher education is dangerous. I have done the research. Here's why. (I used lots of footnotes. Credibility, after all, still mattered.)

I said, Do not force people to disclose. It's awful.

I said, If you want to help disabled people, do not talk down to them, or about them. Don't exert power over them. You are causing harm, even if you, too, are disabled.

I said all of the things I wished I'd said last time but was too afraid to.

Although keeping your disability a secret can be an awful burden, and I wish everyone could share and alleviate that burden, I know they cannot. Those who feel vulnerable should not feel like they are cowards for not disclosing.

When you have a disability that is demonized, ostracized, and scapegoated, you can measure your life as a series of painful encounters. As one surgeon told me, discovering I had bipolar disorder, "I don't want you to have an episode on my table." Reading the TSA PreCheck questions about mental illness made me cry once we left the building.[14] Some pharmacists warily eye mentally disabled people when we pick up our monthly medications. For mentally disabled people, there is so much pain in everyday encounters.

I disclose, however, because I also hold out hope. I put my reputation on the line because if I can convince one more person that mental disability is not something to be feared, I have done good work. I *choose* to disclose to readers, colleagues, and students. I choose to do the work of an activist. And hope, by my actions, I make life a little better for every mentally disabled person, even those who must keep their disability secret.

7

Writing Publicly about Mental Disability

Higher education faculty have recently been urged by their institutions and scholarly organizations to do public writing about their areas of knowledge. For example, in August of 2022, the Modern Language Association (MLA) released guidelines "to help departments, institutions, and faculty members in languages and literatures value and assess public humanities work."[1] By providing a way for departments to assign value to public writing, the MLA encourages faculty to do so. Faculty are interested in writing for the public—the plethora of advice columns and conference workshops on this subject attest to this fact.

Yet many faculty are not prepared for what it means to step into public discourse. There are risks, and there are rewards. Such risks and rewards intensify when you write publicly about any politically contentious, typically private, and emotional subject—such as mental disability or, say, sexual assault.[2] Only *you* can know what those rewards might be for you. You might want to write for the money. The pay for most online publications is poor, but even two hundred dollars here and there can make a difference to a contingent faculty member who is scraping by. You might write for social capital—and you will get some if your piece makes a splash. You might write as a form of activism. This is the main reason I do so—I try to use words to change the world for the better.

But when we write about mental disability for the public, we must also recognize the risks we face. Some disability studies faculty believe all disabled faculty have a duty to publicly disclose their disabilities within the confines of academic conferences. (I discuss this debate in Chapter 6.) I disagree because the risks of disclosure can be severe—to one's reputation and one's career. In this chapter I discuss disclosing in a public forum, which presents different risks. With that in mind, here are some of the things you should consider before diving into the deep end of public discourse when writing about your own mental disability.

The Double Bind of Disclosure

What if you write about being disabled, but no one believes you?

When you write publicly about being disabled, whether mentally disabled in particular or disabled in general, you will face a frustrating double bind: Some readers will not believe you are disabled at all (the Doubter). And some readers will hold your disability against you, using it to discredit your authority as a writer (the Patronizer). I am telling you about this double bind up front because there is no right way to disclose that will shut these ableists down. You will encounter them no matter what.

The Doubter thinks, "You are way too together to be that sick." For example, when I write about being autistic, there is always a Doubter (or five) who will say something like this: "There is no way you're autistic (or "really autistic," whatever that means) if you can write this well." In other words, my skill as a writer belies my disability. For the Doubter, I am not disabled enough for my disability to be real. A Doubter wants you to convince them that you are not a faker. Don't bother. Disabled people are perpetually accused of being fakers, as research shows.[3] In the case of public writing, you must ignore the accusation, even if it's hard.

Then there is the Patronizer. The Patronizer believes your disability is real, sure, but they only see you as disabled. You are no longer a person; you are your disability. Indeed, you are *too* disabled, per the Patronizer. Many Patronizers wrote to me that I was a bad parent, for example, when I published a high-profile piece on depression. One wrote: "I think you're kidding yourself if you think living with someone who oozes unhappiness doesn't have an impact [on your kids]."[4] I mean, I know I do not "ooze unhappiness," but the words stung. A lot.

The Doubter and the Patronizer, together, make up a double bind that every disabled person faces when deciding whether to publicly disclose a disability. This double bind is part of the stigma of mental disability. Either a person does not believe you, and therefore they think you must be exaggerating your disabilities to seek attention. Or they do believe you, and therefore they think you are too disabled to take care of yourself, take care of your family, or do your job.

The stigma against mental disabilities is something you must take seriously before you consider writing publicly about your own disability. If you feel like you have to walk a tightrope to please readers—know that you do not. If you encounter an editor who is a Doubter or a Patronizer—do not write for them. Know that most of your readers are quietly reading your words and are grateful that you wrote them.

Psychic Toll of Writing

Frequently, writing about mental disability can be traumatic. The act of disclosure is difficult, and every single time you write, you are disclosing anew—to a different editor, to a different audience, or about a different aspect of yourself. The act of writing about something hard is also traumatic. The point is, writing about hard stuff takes a psychic toll, and you need to be prepared for that.

I started writing publicly about mental disability back in 2014 when I began my monthly column "Life of the Mind Interrupted" with *The Chronicle of Higher Education*. The column ran for three years, and the column name (and much of the work) became my 2017 book of the same title.[5] Writing a column month after month on mental illness and disability was hard work. Not because there wasn't much to say—there was—but because, with every column I wrote, I had to give a little bit of myself to the world.

Later, for two years, I wrote a column titled "Mom Interrupted" for the magazine *Catapult* about being a neurodivergent mom with neurodivergent kids.[6] From 2018 to 2020 I wrote these essays, and they are, in my opinion, some of my very best writing. But in order to do the writing for *Catapult*, I had to give even more of myself than I did for my *Chronicle* column. The essays drained a lot of my mental and emotional energy. (Luckily, my editor was very understanding, and she allowed me time to recover between essays.)

Frequently, telling your stories about mental disability will drain you. The best advice I can give you is this: You must plan for the draining and give yourself time to recover. Your assignment might be twelve hundred words, but the toll may be far greater than the word count. You will struggle as you write the hard thing. You will struggle as you work with an editor. And then, the day your piece is published, you will struggle again when the public consumes your work. If you are aware, now, of that psychic toll, then you can plan for it.

Professional Consequences of Disclosure

Another risk of writing publicly about mental disability is that there may be negative professional and personal consequences that come along with disclosing your disability. Mental disabilities are stigmatized in our society, especially in higher education. Depending on your situation (work, family, and so on), you might not feel safe disclosing your own disability in a public fashion. You need to think hard about whether you should disclose that you have a mental disability. And even if you do disclose, you should then think about whether you should disclose your specific diagnosis.

There are benefits to disclosing. These include increased writerly credibility—if you are a disabled person who is writing about disability, disclosing lets you speak from a position of experience, like this: "I know what it is like to mask as an autistic person because I am autistic."

But the risks, ironically, also have to do with credibility. Mentally disabled people are often considered untrustworthy witnesses of our own experiences. That is, our memories are not trustworthy because our minds are not trustworthy. Therefore, in readers' minds, we cannot be counted on to tell our own stories properly.

This credibility risk/benefit problem is another manifestation of the double bind I mentioned earlier in this chapter: If you do not disclose your mental disability, you lose credibility because you are writing about something you have no experience with. If you do disclose, then you lose credibility because you have a broken brain (no, not really) and are therefore unreliable.

I did not publicly disclose my mental disability until after I left full-time university employment, because I worked in a contingent position and my job was constantly insecure. Your position might be secure, and your workplace might be very supportive. But if your job is contingent, your position is insecure, and/or your institution is unsupportive of your public writing, you should consider the consequences of disclosing and also of writing online—you not only have to worry about the response at your institution, but also about the response of the public.

Public Response

The public response to my writing, and to any writing about mental disability, is often passionate—positively and negatively. Rarely is the response tepid: everyone seems to have an opinion about mental illness, neurodiversity, disability, and accessibility. When you wade into these waters, you will not be swimming alone.

You will likely receive private messages; most of them will probably be positive. After I started writing on mental health and higher education, I began receiving lots of messages from others in the academy who were, or had been, in a similar position to mine. Some of these emails thanked me for writing what others did not feel safe saying, or for doing the work I do. Today, I still receive these messages when I publish essays on mental disability, and I really enjoy receiving them. Many of the people who have contacted me over the years have become my friends.

Some pieces will bring bigger reactions than others, and you never know which piece will do it. This unpredictability is part of the psychic toll. The bigger the splash, the more public scrutiny your writing will receive—positive and negative. I usually receive about 95 percent supportive feedback and only 5 percent criticism. But there is definitely criticism. Fortunately, much of it is constructive. For example, recently someone wrote a letter to the editor of the *Chronicle of Higher Education* taking issue with a recent piece I had written. Here's the thing: I was happy that someone had taken the time to read my piece, engage with it, and write a letter about it. And I was delighted that the magazine chose to publish a letter about my piece. That is flattering. Really. And I do not mind criticism of my writing—I learn from others who take the time to point out places where I could have done better.

But some criticism is not so civilized. There are trolls, so many trolls, especially on social media. If you write for the public, you will want to share your work for others to read. Social media, right now, is the best way to do so. But you will get random trolls bagging on your work, especially if you write something that resonates with a lot of people. Those trolls can hit you hard in your soft places, especially if you wrote about something risky.

Some responses are vile attacks. They have attacked my parenting (see above), my teaching, my everything. I receive tweets, direct messages, Facebook messages and posts, and emails targeting everything

I hold dear. You also must consider how your institution will react if you write something that causes a larger negative backlash—even if the backlash is from a wacky fringe group. Will they stand by you?

Tressie McMillan Cottom has written best on this subject. She points to how race, gender, and employment status matter when assessing the public response to engaging in public writing as an academic: "Individuals experience microcelebrity and attention [from public engagement] differently relative to the status groups in which they are embedded. With greater publics and attention, one's social location becomes more salient to the risks and returns to attention."[7] Furthermore, she writes— and she would know—that universities are "woefully underprepared . . . to deal with the reality of public scholarship, public intellectuals, or public engagement."[8] I recommend reading her writing on the subject in its entirety ("Everything But The Burden: Publics, Public Scholarship, And Institutions"), to get a sense of how to discover what support you can expect from your institution. They want the positive publicity you generate, but will they stand by you if things get hard? She provides instructions for how to find out.

Emotional Labor of Responding

If you write for the public and receive responses, some of those responses will be more than just praise or criticism. Some readers will write to you because they see you as a source of support and advice about mental disability. When I first started receiving these messages, I felt it was my duty to reply to any message asking for help or advice. I knew that I was not qualified to offer mental health advice, so I did not give it. But I did believe that the person who had read my work deserved a caring response from me. Thus, I frequently offered an ear to total strangers on the internet who just wanted someone to talk to. At first, I spent a lot of energy replying to every stranger whose message landed in my inbox, and I felt sapped after every reply. Do not do what I did. Here's some advice for how to respond to the various types of messages you will likely receive.

Professional advice queries. These are the types of messages I receive most frequently: "I am an associate chair of a department and would like to educate my faculty about mental health. What should I do?" To these queries, I write a short, kind email wishing the person well, and then I direct them to my written work or offer to facilitate a workshop (for pay). You could offer to give a webinar or point them to other writing you have done.

Nonemergency mental health advice. The second most common messages I receive from readers about mental health are those who just want to talk about their own struggles. I reply with a short, kind email wishing the person well. Then I tell them I am not a mental health professional, and I advise them to seek the services of one. I do not get engaged in a chat with a stranger about their mental health.

Immediate crisis. Very rarely, a person will write to me in an immediate crisis situation. I tell them to call 911 (or the emergency number in their country if they are not in the United States). I do not waste time with any other words. I am very direct: "You are in a medical crisis. Call 911 or a hotline right now." If a person is reaching out to a stranger on the internet because they are contemplating suicide, they feel alone and need help. If they try to engage in a conversation about why they do not need to call 911, or if they try to tell me that 911 is an overreaction to suicidal ideation, I do not engage. I simply repeat what I wrote above. This person is in a medical crisis, and they need to call 911 or a suicide hotline, not me. Fortunately, crises like these have only happened a few times. They are very stressful, as you can imagine.

If You Are Ready to Get Started

If writing for the public appeals to you, the first step is to set yourself up for success by learning how to join the professional community of public writers. You need to professionalize.

Learn the skills. First, you pitch. Then, you receive an acceptance or a rejection. Then you write, usually on a very tight deadline. Then you interact with an editor—who may accept your piece or "kill" it. Then your piece is published, and you are expected to publicize it (on social media). How do you do all of these things? You likely have not been taught how to write for the public, so you have to teach yourself. For example, you can learn from experts how to write a pitch—Kelly J. Baker, a mentally disabled author and former editor of multiple difference magazines, has taught public writing workshops and provides instructions, on her website (kellyjbaker.com), for how to pitch.[9]

Build a community. Before you step into public writing about mental disability, build a community of other writers like you. I have a great community of disabled writers that I built using social media. We help each other out in a variety of ways. For example, we know which editors are supportive of our work, and which are not. When one of us publishes something, we boost one another's work. We stand up for one another when trolls come around.

After you write and publish your first piece, or before you even do so, you might decide you do not want to be a public writer at all. You might find it tempting to add your voice to the debates about mental disability, but you might also find that you do not want to risk disclosure or the possibility of negative attacks. Public writing might just feel overwhelming. In the end, it is your choice. You have no duty to disclose or to debate publicly. No one should feel pressured to do so.

8

Writing Depression

Depression—and all mental disabilities—is notoriously difficult to write about. William Styron, in his memoir *Darkness Visible,* describes the difficulty of writing about depression: "Since antiquity—in the tortured lament of Job, in the choruses of Sophocles and Aeschylus—chroniclers of the human spirit have been wrestling with a vocabulary that might give proper expression to the desolation of melancholia."[1] To make matters more difficult, it is extremely hard to write while you are depressed or riddled with anxiety. Research shows that depression causes loss of both executive function and memory. Doing any coherent writing while depressed, as any writer with depression will tell you, is nearly impossible. The best we can do is write badly. But sometimes that is enough.

Why Write When You're Depressed?

When you are depressed, you frequently do not remember details when you come out of it. Research shows that depression affects brain function, including the making of memories.[2] After I gave birth to my second child in 2011, I suffered from terrible postpartum depression. It took months to heal. The worst part? I remember very little from the first three months of my son's life. I see the photographs from that time, and I do not even remember them being taken. There are people in them I do not recognize. Having this blank spot in my memory is a horribly disorienting feeling, and I also feel deep grief. After that period of my life, I decided I would start writing depression.

I believe it is crucial to write while we are depressed, at the very least to preserve these memories we would otherwise lose. It is your choice whether to share what you write. After all, you will likely believe that it is trash. (When one is depressed, one believes everything is trash.) But, perhaps later when you are no longer depressed, you may choose to share your writing. And if you do share your writing, your words can combat stigma by giving an inside look into something few people see. You will welcome outsiders into depression. And when you do so, you normalize depression, removing the shame associated with it and other mental disabilities.

But you may choose never to share your writing, and that's okay. You may only want to capture what you feel in the depressed moment so that you can clarify the experience for yourself, later. There is great value in writing depression only for yourself.

I first wrote about depression many years ago. I did so to preserve memories; I wanted to have a view into my state of mind later. At the time I was depressed, I knew that I would forget what I was thinking and feeling once I had healed.

Ever since that first time, I have tried to write at least once during every bout of depression. My most recent serious depression came in 2019.

Here's what I wrote.

Depression, The Essay[3]

Today, I am painfully, horribly, depressed.

I was also depressed yesterday, and the day before. And last week. And the week before. And last month. Likely the month before, and the month before that. I don't recall much prior because the rest is covered in fog.

When you are depressed, much is covered in fog.

When you are depressed, you—I—don't want to write. I decided to write about this bout of depression, though. I am consoling myself with one statement I'm repeating over and over, this one: You can delete this tomorrow. If you hate it, if you are embarrassed, if it is a stinking pile of garbage words you can delete it whenever you want to.

When you are depressed, you think everything you do is garbage.

When you are depressed, it is easier to write in the second person than the first person because it's hard to talk about yourself.

But I'll try.

Even though I'm depressed, I've been telling everyone that I have the flu. That way, I don't have to talk to people because talking to people, seeing people, is unbearable. Having the flu also gives me an excuse to lie in bed at odd hours.

At the same time, for the sake of my children, I'm getting up each morning at six a.m. I'm getting dressed, even putting on makeup to brighten my eyes. My eyes, when I look in the mirror, appear so dull. In fact, my new dedication to makeup has caught the interest of both of my sons, to the point that they've wandered into my bathroom in curiosity to watch me do it, asking me questions about it.

I learned a new word today, one I was surprised I didn't already know. "Anhedonia." I love this word. If you took Latin, or are fascinated by words, you will decipher what it means.

"Hedonist." There's a word you might already know.

An-hedon-ia.

I'm in a state of anhedonia, my doctor told me, where the things that used to cause me pleasure bring me no pleasure. Nothing makes me happy. Food isn't enjoyable. Nothing is enjoyable.

Things don't make me sad necessarily. No, I'm in a state of suspended pointlessness. It's torture.

Earlier today, I decided to dedicate myself to "tiny tasks." Small wins, as my friend Ariane calls them. I will not try to climb any mountains. I just want to check some things off of my to-do list because my to-do list is so long it's making me more depressed. So, this morning, I did a thing. It was great.

So I did another thing. And it has become—I cannot state this in words strong enough—terrible. Here's what happened: while doing a cursory book order for the small press I run, I discovered, by accident, that one of the books that our press publishes had been taken out of the catalog by our distributor—for no reason, just an error, a glitch.

In short, what this glitch means is that no one can purchase this particular book anywhere in the world.

And the hell of it is that no one at the press knew about it until I tried to place that book order. Who knows how long the book has been, essentially, out of print?

And why didn't we know about it? The answer is simple: because I've been depressed. It's my fault. I blame myself for not noticing sooner, for not scanning the sales sheets closely enough. Maybe I should blame the distributor, whose fault it is for mistakenly killing the distribution. But I blame me for not keeping proper tabs on things. That's my job. Big distributors make mistakes. People like me need to pay attention.

And I can't. Pay. Attention. That's what it means to be depressed. There isn't any currency with which to make those payments.

I have no resources. I'm fresh out.

One month of sales of one of our bestselling titles. Gone. And it's my fault.

So now I have to call the distributor to fix the problem. I have to argue with a human. My resources are now in the negative. Worse, I'm still waiting on their fix to come through. The book is still in limbo. I can't bear the thought of this problem. I want to weep.

The tiny task has become not just any mountain. It's Everest.

I set it aside even though it is still haunting me. I shove it aside, or I will not be able to do anything else.

I take on another tiny task. A simple email newsletter. I write it, I keep it short and lovely. I proof it. I send it to our small press's entire email list. And then, when I receive my copy of it, there is an ugly, awful, disgusting typo that I missed. So awful. So ugly. I can't even bear it.

I still can't bear it. The thought of that typo. I only had the one small job to do. And I couldn't even do that right.

I'm a failure at everything I touch. I can't fix big problems. I can't fix small ones. I can't even write properly—as I reread what I've written here, it sounds so stupid and terrible. I'm resisting deleting it. I'm resisting, but it is so hard.

After the newsletter, I call my doctor. She is worried. So she prescribes more medicine to help. I walk to the pharmacy to pick up the prescription. Then I walk home. Except when I get home, my car isn't here. That's when I realize that I didn't walk to the pharmacy. I drove, and then I forgot my car at the pharmacy.

My brain isn't working. I've accepted that. Honestly, I can't explain to you how much my brain isn't working except to tell you this story, the story about how during the short trip to the pharmacy to pick up medicine to help me stop being depressed I completely forgot that I had an automobile.

When I arrive home, and realize I forgot it, I don't have the energy to go back and get it. I leave it there for the rest of the day. I call my husband crying, telling him about the book being killed from distribution, about the typo. I tell him about leaving my car. I can't stop crying. I don't know how to stop.

The worst part is that I know how ridiculous all of this sounds. That's why writing these words is so hard. I know. I know. I know. This is not the first time I've been depressed. I'm in my midforties. I have bipolar disorder. I've been depressed many times. And every time, it's so horrible. Every time, when my husband hugs me, wrapping me in our bedspread and squeezing the tears out like I'm a lemon, I wonder why he stays with me year after year, when he knows that days (weeks, months) like this will always come again.

I'm writing these words even though I know they are self-indulgent, and boring, and embarrassing, and garbage. Even though I sound weak and sad and pathetic. I'm going to write them, and I'm going to share them.

Because if you are out there, and you are like me, in pain so much pain, and the sun makes you cry instead of making you feel warm, and food tastes like sawdust, and you always shake with chills no matter how much you bundle up or how many covers you put on your bed, and everything you touch just rots—I want you to know that I feel that way too, despite what I look like on the outside.

If all we show is a glossy surface, then we all suffer even more. My surface seems glossy, but it isn't real. These words are what is real. I'm depressed, and it hurts.

The Email from Brad

The bout of depression I wrote about above came during the winter holidays of 2018. At the time I didn't notice I was depressed because the holidays always hit me hard emotionally. And then, in February of 2019, my father-in-law died, and you are supposed to be sad when someone dies, so my sadness masked my depression a while longer. A few weeks after that, my child was sick with pneumonia for weeks; I could not think about anything while he slept next to me because I was counting each of his labored inhalations. I believed I was merely sleep-deprived and worried, not depressed.

By the time late March rolled around, I had so many excuses for feeling poorly that I never considered I might be depressed, and those excuses hurt my ability to get medical care. But finally I figured it out. That was when I decided to start writing about being depressed, even though the last thing I wanted to do was write anything.

I wrote about depression a lot in March. I could not think of anything else to write about (because I was depressed). Then I published a little of what I wrote, as the essay you just read above, on my website.

Sometimes, I get emails from companies that want me to feature sponsored content on my site. Most of these emails I just delete because they are obviously not targeted at me personally. But after I published this latest essay, I received one email that I could not ignore, even though I should have.

The salutation began "Dear Katie," like we were friends, and then the writer explained why he had contacted me: "I was doing some digging on depression-related articles . . . " He then pointed to my recent essay. Regarding his own website, he wrote, "Our readers wanted more inspirational and actionable self-development content, and we thought your readers might enjoy it too." I snorted, literally, when I read the words "inspirational" and "actionable." Then he included a request for me to post his, apparently, more inspirational and actionable web copy about depression.

I deleted the email.

Then I undeleted it and saved it, stewing on it. I thought about inspiration porn, the term coined by Stella Young, the late Australian disability activist.[4] Inspiration porn is a term to describe media portrayals of disabled people used to generate feelings of sentimentality or pity in abled people or to send an uplifting message to abled people. "Look, this kid with one leg can run a 5K. You, abled person, can do it too!" One of the many problems with inspiration porn is that it is so pervasive and normalized that the standard normate expectation of disability stories is that they "inspire." In other words, if your disability story is not sentimental or uplifting, publishers don't want to publish it, and many readers don't want to read it.

Thus, if you are a disabled writer telling a story about your disability, the standard normate expectation requires an uplifting story about you overcoming your disability. You *must* find a way to magically heal your body or mind and stop being disabled altogether, at least metaphorically, if not actually.

When I read the email from the spammy guy asking if he could post inspirational nonsense on my blog after reading about my soul-destroying depression, I wanted to write him a cuss-laden reply about where he could stick his sponsored content. But I did not. What a waste of time that would be. I could be yelling at a bot. Worse, I could be yelling at some guy named Brad who actually wanted to collaborate with me on invigorating mental health listicles.

Instead, I started thinking about the writing I have done on depression over the years, and then I realized this: The suffering is part of my story, but people are constantly trying to take it away. Brad is just the most recent person who strutted into my space, telling me my story is wrong. And Brad definitely did not deserve my time.

Our Stories Are Ours

Every time I publish an essay about being disabled and someone writes comments like, "You seem totally normal to me" or "I don't see you as disabled, just different," they are taking away my story. I am disabled. A reader might wish to see me differently, but why? This language is undermining and counterproductive. It feeds into the feelings of worthlessness and invisibility that already make it hard to write about disability topics and reinforce abled norms. The fact is, I am not totally normal, and telling me that I seem so is not a compliment—it is erasure.

I believe that many normates, in the end, are uncomfortable with disability stories that do not have tidy, inspirational endings. To wit: I will never "get better" from bipolar disorder. I will never overcome it. I will be depressed sometimes, hopefully less depressed than I was in the spring of 2019 (because hopefully I will notice sooner). I will have upswings in mood as well, not full-blown mania, because I take medicine, which I love, and it works. But the fact is, there is no cure.

I am autistic. There is no cure. I don't *want* a cure. Autistic is who I am, and cure-based narratives, fictional and nonfictional, tell me that I am made wrong. I'm fortunate enough to know that I am not. But there are others who aren't as self-certain as I am, and I worry for them.

A glance at popular narratives bears out my observation about cures: At the end of the film *A Beautiful Mind*, mathematician John Nash, who has schizophrenia, "gets better" and wins a Nobel Prize as well (although Nash's actual life story is not at all so tidy).[5] In the Marvel film *Captain America: Civil War*, James Rhodes ("War Machine") falls and becomes paraplegic from a spinal injury. But at the end, he is able to walk using technology from Tony Stark ("Iron Man").[6]

Sometimes mentally disabled people suffer. Sometimes living hurts, a lot. But what we are doing with this living is merely being human. Sometimes humans suffer. Inclusion means that disabled people are recognized as full and complete people and that our communities embrace stories that do not toe the inspiration line. We get to tell our own stories, our way. Fortunately, the publishing industry is gradually becoming more accepting of disability stories that challenge the inspiration narrative.[7]

If disabled people are writing for the public, it can be hard to reject normate expectations of disability stories—disability porn—but we must do so in order to write freely and to have the confidence to share our darkest experiences. If we are writing for ourselves, we also must be careful of these social norms that might have crept inside us. When we are writing depression, the depression is ours, and we owe it to ourselves, to our memories, to put the full truth on the page.

Part II

Teaching with Mental Health in Mind

9

"The Darkness That Is Plaguing Our University"

The terrible email from the university chancellor came on a Sunday afternoon in October of 2021. At the time, I thought it was strange that the chancellor would send an email blast to the entire university on a Sunday. But the email's opening explained its arrival day: "Today, on World Mental Health Day, we are taking a moment to acknowledge and reflect on the seriousness of mental health illness and the challenges we face as we wrestle with the stress and pressures of our world today."[1] World Mental Health Day fell on a Sunday. That made sense.

But then the email continued, moving from a worldwide day of recognition to something more serious: "We are in the middle of a mental health crisis, both on our campus and across our nation." Finally, I thought, campus leadership was acknowledging the campus mental health crisis rather than sweeping it under the rug.[2] As the chancellor's email continued, my chest tightened with fear: "We are aware that college-aged students carry an increased risk of suicide. This crisis has directly impacted members of our community—especially with the passing of two students on campus in the past month." Shocked, I could not believe that I had not heard anything about two students dying by suicide so recently on our campus. How did this news not make it to my ear? Suicide is not a *wow that is so sad* thing to me. It's personal. The fact that I hadn't heard meant that things had been kept quiet.

I knew that the administration needed to tread carefully with the news. One reason schools keep student suicide quiet is because of suicide contagion, also called the "Werther Effect," which can be caused by media attention given to those who have died by suicide.[3] Another reason is because of the taboo that shrouds mental health struggles, especially death by suicide. Suicide and depression are stigmatized and shameful.

After the chancellor's letter went public, news outlets scrambled to cover our campus tragedies. NBC News interviewed students, who provided gut-wrenching observations about the campus mental health climate: "'Our hearts are shattered,' said Kendra Randle, a junior." Later in the interview, Randle continued, "After we spend time mourning, we need to figure out solutions to this darkness that is plaguing our university."[4]

Searching for Answers

After receiving the chancellor's email, I began to research the students' deaths. It was a struggle to learn more details—the news reports merely regurgitated the chancellor's email.[5] Most of the news reports I found mentioned only the death and attempted suicide that occurred the October weekend when the email was sent. What about the second death that the chancellor reported in his email? I kept digging through the news, trying to get to a truth that seemed to be too hard to find. Eventually, I found one report where the writer had thoroughly dug through our campus police log and reported that another student died by suicide on September 4, 2021, and another attempted on September 22.[6]

Desperate for more information I, too, turned to the police log—a website open to the public—which tracks not just stolen bicycles and laptops, but also mental health events.[7] I researched five weeks of data that occurred after the chancellor's email in October. As I scrolled through the log, I looked for anything related to mental health. I found three types of items. First, I found welfare checks. A welfare check is a police action taken when a worried family member or friend asks the police to come to a person's home to make sure they are safe. The most common cause for welfare checks among young people is concern for mental health safety.[8] Across the five weeks I studied, I found seventeen welfare checks. I also found seven voluntary and one involuntary committal to inpatient psychiatric care. Nearly all of these events occurred in student residence halls.

Thus, in just over a month after the chancellor declared a mental health crisis on campus, we had twenty-five police-involved mental health events. These bare records tell a dark story about our community and the mental health of our students. First, that is a lot of police involvement in student mental health crises. Do you recall, when you were a teenager or a college student, what it took for you to call the police for help? Do you recall the sorts of crises that we believed, in our youthful hubris, we were capable of handling on our own? We were always in over our heads, sometimes in dire situations; we just didn't know it. Each of these calls on the police log represents a moment so dire that the only thing a panicked college kid could think to do was call the police, the very last resort for most young people. By that same logic, each call we see on the log represents many mental health crises for which the police were not called. The log represents the tip of a very large iceberg.

What I have learned through my research is this: student deaths by suicide are a nationwide epidemic. The Healthy Minds Study in 2020 reported that 39 percent of students screened positive for depression (major and moderate) and 13 percent for suicidal ideation.[9] At schools across the country, our students are dying. In thirteen months spanning 2021 and 2022, Stanford University had thirteen students die by suicide, a crisis by any standard. The highest profile of the deaths was that of Katie Meyer, who served as captain and goalkeeper of Stanford's soccer team, which won the NCAA championship in 2019. She died in March of 2022.[10] Closer to home, during the 2022–2023 school year, North Carolina State University (Raleigh, North Carolina) has had seven students die by suicide.[11] NC State is only twenty minutes down the road from Chapel Hill.

Intersections of Race and Mental Health Struggles

The campus mental health crisis is affecting students differently depending on their race and ethnicity, and how we approach taking care of our students must take race and ethnicity into account. In a study published in 2021, researchers found that 17 percent of the Black students they interviewed screened positive for suicide risk.[12] But of this group, 66 percent were *not* receiving mental health services.[13] The researchers found that four main barriers prevented these students from seeking help: they perceived their mental health struggles weren't that bad, they didn't have time, they felt fear and stigma, and they worried about money.[14]

Of note, however, Black students found fear and stigma to be greater barriers than (white) college students in past studies. Research showed that 55 percent of Black students reported that fear and stigma stopped them from seeking help.[15] The researchers noted that "given the historical maltreatment of Blacks in the U.S. by medical providers and research studies documenting the prevalence of stigma related to [mental health care] among Black adults and families, fear/stigma as a primary barrier to [mental health care] is not surprising."[16] What this research shows is that to reach Black students struggling with their mental health, colleges need to tailor their approach to Black students to take this heightened stigma into account.

The Asian American Psychological Association reports that Asian American college students are more likely than white students to have had suicidal ideation and to attempt suicide.[17] These high rates of suicide among Asian American students have led to suicide crises on various campuses, including Cornell and MIT. Reported by Jenn Fang at *Reappropriate*, from 2000–2015, "MIT's suicide rate was 29.1 per 100,000 Asian American students. This is not only nearly four times the overall national average and three times the average for the school, but also more than twice the national average for college-aged Asian Americans."[18] At Cornell, Fang reported, 61 percent of on-campus deaths by suicide in the decade between 1996 and 2006 were Asian American students. In response to its Asian American suicide crisis, Cornell addressed the issue directly when it "committed to genuinely prioritize this issue with specific regard to Asian American students." For example, it created an Asian and Asian American Center on campus to support this student group. Few schools, though, are willing to handle the intersection of race and mental health as proactively as Cornell did.

The takeaway is this: each student population must be met on its own terms. Race, ethnicity, and other identity factors put students at risk of mental disability and suicide in different ways. But for decades, campuses have struggled to keep up with students' needs, and matters are only getting worse.

Understaffed Campus Counseling

The students' deaths at UNC, at NC State, and on other campuses correlate with a lack of campus support for the high rates of students' anxiety and depression. Higher education institutions are scrambling to understand what "support" means to a student who is facing mental health struggles. Most, but not all, students who come to college leave behind a familiar support structure to land in a place that provides very little support at all. When students arrive on campus, institutions must presume that all of them are going through an emotional shock to some degree. Some students will settle easily into new support systems. Students from vulnerable groups, such as those with mental disabilities, will have a harder time doing so.

On-campus counseling centers are staffed by wonderful and generous workers, but most centers have been long understaffed and unable to adequately serve their student communities. Recently, instead of hiring more workers, institutions have begun outsourcing their counseling services to third-party teletherapy services like UWill (uwill.com), which claims it "incorporates cutting edge technologies that facilitate best-in-class video and message-based counseling."[19] Top universities have contracted with this service, including the University of Maryland at College Park, Boston College, the University of North Carolina at Chapel Hill (my own institution, who hired them in 2019), and the entire University of Massachusetts system. A similar service, Timely.md, has clients that include Duke University, the University of Virginia, and Middlebury College. In other words, these outsourced telehealth therapy services are no longer on the fringe of college counseling services. On the contrary, institutions have been overwhelmed with counseling needs for years, and they adopted remote telehealth services to solve the problem.

Do these services meet student needs? Maybe. Nicole Ruzek, director of Counseling and Psychological Services at the University of Virginia, told *Inside Higher Ed* that "the switch to more virtual mental health resources has opened up access for students from families or cultural backgrounds that typically don't seek mental health help," which is a definite benefit.[20] But other campus leaders report that "students are split between wanting in-person or virtual mental health services."

Another key problem with the traditional counseling model, whether virtual or in person, is that it puts the burden on the student to reach out for help in the first place—it is a passive service. When you are depressed, stressed out, or anxious, passive services are difficult to access. You are either too depressed to get out of bed or too anxious to take the time to make an appointment. In addition to providing traditional counseling, if institutions want to reach all students in need, they must put in place active support. But these online services could be transformed into active support. For example, institutions could put in place check-ins through the online services that they have contracted with; a counselor on the app would message each student directly, asking how they are doing. If a student does not reply, or replies in a concerning way, a message goes to the campus counseling system to check on that student.

Part of the burden of student care falls heavily on certain members of the faculty, whom I call "front-line faculty."[21] These are the faculty whom students turn to because they are the easiest for students to form relationships with—their first-year writing professors, the professors who teach the small sections of large lectures, and so on. Front-line faculty have close contact with students and are therefore in a position to notice—and do something about—students' mental health struggles. Front-line faculty are the people whom students turn to first when they are struggling, so they bear an immense emotional burden. Despite this work, front-line faculty do not receive adequate support for the work they do. Furthermore, faculty on the front lines tend to be the most vulnerable in higher education because of marginalized status (women of color, white women, disabled people, LGBTQI+, family caregivers, and so on) and lack of job security from working contingent positions. Thus, a large part of the burden of student caretaking has been passed to the most vulnerable faculty on campus. (I discuss front-line faculty in detail in Chapter 13.)

Depression, Students, and Stigma

The day I dug through the police logs at UNC, I wondered whether it would help if the university made the information that I painstakingly gathered more accessible to the public. Right now, in the way the logs are presented, these mental health interventions are difficult to find. The site is very low-tech, and it is not keyword searchable. If one wanted to find out just how much of a mental health crisis UNC was facing, it would take hours and hours of research. The difficulty of accessing this data keeps mental health struggles in the shadows and maintains the stigma against mental disability. The chancellor wrote that we were in a mental health crisis. But what exactly did that mean? It was far too difficult for me to find out what I did, and I definitely did not find out everything. That would be impossible. There is an immense space for intervention between doing nothing and calling the police, which means that what I found in the police log represents only a small corner of the campus mental health picture.

(Ideally students would not have to call the police for a mental health intervention. Having police perform mental health care is itself a public health problem. Nearly 25 percent of people killed by police had a "known mental illness."[22] Unfortunately, the project of separating policing and mental health is beyond the scope of this book.)

Perhaps a student called the outsourced mental health hotline and received adequate nonpolice aid.[23] Perhaps a student's roommate or friend helped them through a dark night. According to the Healthy Minds Study Fall 2020 Data Report (HMS), 14 percent of students sought mental health support from their roommates and 40 percent from other friends.[24] A student is lucky if they have friends whom they can trust with their mental health struggles. Perhaps a student gutted it out alone. The HMS reported many barriers to students seeking help, including these: 17 percent because help was too expensive, 18 percent because there was not enough time, 13 percent because they were not sure where to go, 7 percent because they could not get an appointment, and 4 percent because the service providers "didn't understand" the student.

Some students avoid seeking help, however, because they feel ashamed to share their pain with anyone else. Students understand the stigma against seeking mental health care. The HMS reported that 45 percent of students agreed with this statement: "Most people would think less of someone who has received mental health treatment." When nearly half of our students believe that most people stigmatize the seeking of mental health care, it is not surprising that they would avoid seeking it. Individuals struggling with their mental health should not feel shame. There is nothing shameful about it. Nevertheless, in our ableist society, the stigma of mental disability leads to shame about anything to do with mental health.

Students have another good reason to keep information about mental health struggles from their fellow students and professors. There is a not-insignificant chance that an institution will force a student out of school, as journalist Katie J. M. Baker reports in a piece about such practices.[25] Baker writes that "dozens of current or recent students at colleges and universities across the country . . . were punished for seeking [mental health] help: kicked out of campus housing with nowhere else to go, abruptly forced to withdraw from school and even involuntarily committed to psychiatric wards."[26] Author Esmé Weijun Wang recounts just such an experience about being forced out of Yale: "Rather than receiving help, mentally ill students are frequently, as I was, pressured into leaving—or ordered to leave—by the schools that once welcomed them."[27] There are similar cases across the country, including at Stanford University, where six students sued the school in 2018, "arguing they were forced to put their education on hold for months or a year because they had told university officials about their mental health problems."[28] Worse, in the same case, "one student, cited anonymously in the litigation, said that after she reported having suicidal thoughts, Stanford threatened to expel her if she did not take a year-long leave of absence." Research shows that "placing a student struggling with mental health on medical leave, a policy found on many college campuses, does not necessarily facilitate recovery."[29] On the contrary, these policies "may have the opposite of their intended effect: permitting a college's most vulnerable students to fall through the cracks."[30] Thus, students not only have stigma to fear, but the loss of their diplomas.

Seeking help for suicidal thoughts in particular can be difficult because suicide itself carries a mark of shame in our society. First, there is the shame that families and friends of the dead experience. Research shows that "unlike other modes of death, suicide is stigmatized, despite recent valiant strides to destigmatize mental illness and suicide."[31] Bereaved people find it "difficult to talk to others about their loss because others often feel uncomfortable talking about the suicide. This can leave the bereaved feeling isolated." They also feel a "need to conceal the cause of death." This suicide-related shame is externally induced, and we must, as a society and as higher education communities, work to remove it if we hope to prevent suicide in the future. Even the language "committed suicide" hearkens back to a time when suicide was a crime that a person committed, as one commits larceny or murder. In 1964, nine states still had suicide listed as a crime in their statute books (although the crime was rarely prosecuted against suicide survivors).[32] Crimes are shameful, and so is the language of criminality. A quick way to begin to battle stigma is to change how you talk about suicide. Stop using the word "commit," and instead say that someone "died by suicide." The word "commit" has been the norm for a long time; changing how we speak about suicide can be a hard habit to break. But it is important that we do so: how we talk about suicide, depression, and mental disability affects how we treat those affected by suicide, depression, and mental disability.

What Can Institutions Do?

Institutions must do more to support student mental health. They can start by recognizing just how much help students need—and how bad things are. On the Tuesday following the chancellor's email, UNC–Chapel Hill canceled classes, declaring it a "Wellness Day"—not on Monday, which many found odd. The Undergraduate Student Government and the Graduate and Professional Student Government issued a joint letter on Sunday requesting a "break from instruction from Monday, Oct. 11 through the end of day Tuesday, Oct. 12 to allow the Carolina community time to grieve and seek out essential mental health resources."[33] Their request went unheeded. The student body president at the time, Lamar Richards, wrote on social media, "If you are a professor requiring a class to meet tomorrow [Monday] you are part of the problem. We are not machines with on and off switches . . . We are students and we need a break."[34]

Students do, indeed, need a break. Faculty don't have to look hard to see the consequences of the mental health crisis, including more student absences, poor student work, and more late work.[35] The pandemic might have brought this crisis to a head, but it has been building for years. And now the pandemic has left a wide and powerful wake, and our students may take years to recover. It is possible, too, that our students have been changed forever, and therefore our institutions must change with them. Let's use this opportunity to change for the better.

The problem with the stigma that shrouds depression and suicide is that it causes those who are struggling to believe they must suffer in silence. The job of institutions, and of faculty, is to eradicate that stigma. We can bring in campus speakers to share their stories of depression and attempted suicide to spark conversations. We can put genuine, supportive language on our syllabi. If faculty are willing to share their stories, we should pay them to speak and host question-and-answer sessions with them. All of these steps will help eradicate the stigma of mental health struggles on campus, pushing us further toward the goal of a truly neurodiverse and anti-ableist environment, where students with depression and other mental health struggles will emerge, finally, from the shadows. All of this work will normalize seeking help in times of crisis.

10

Rigor Angst

The pandemic caused an awakening to student mental health. Some faculty embraced it and changed their teaching to address their new knowledge. Others did not. In the past, I always believed that I taught accessibly. After the awakening post-COVID, I realized how much more I could do to make my learning accessible for my students. I reevaluated every assignment in my courses, every task, every policy. This reevaluation has become an ongoing part of my pedagogy because I do not believe that learning and the accommodation of our students' mental health struggles are exclusive of one another.

As I had this big realization and began reworking my courses, I did not realize that I was stumbling into the debate over academic "rigor," an issue that has long been a higher education bogeyman. For example, there was a 2016 debate about improving student learning by transforming lecture-based courses into ones that include active learning, based on research that shows that lectures are ineffective. Lecture-defenders howled in protest, arguing that the lecture model must be preserved because "it has endured for hundreds of years for good reason: It works."[1] (They did not say why or how.) If we fail to preserve the lecture model, they argued, we will be contributing to "the erosion of educational standards and let students off the hook for their own learning." In summary, lecture-defenders argued that because something they love has worked (supposedly) for centuries, professors should keep at it—even in the face of research indicating that lectures do not, in fact, work.[2] Instead of holding themselves, as teachers, accountable for their students' learning, the lecture-defenders blame students for failing to learn, preferring to keep students on the "hook," so to speak, if they fail. Otherwise, we go too easy on them, and courses lose their "rigor."[3]

In this context, when I took a firm position that good education and course design to support student mental health could exist side by side, I unwittingly took a side in the rigor debate—the side against rigor. Empathetic course policies like mine coddled students; an empathetic teaching style like mine let them off the so-called hook.

As I looked more into the rigor debate, however, especially at the loud defenses of rigor, what I kept seeing was fear on the part of teachers— what I call "rigor angst." Rigor angst is the fear, held by a professor or administrator, that a curriculum will not be difficult enough to meet the academic standards of a particular institution, department, or course.

The problem with rigor angst, and the ironically unrigorous defenses of "rigor" that it incites, is that it puts our students' mental health and education at risk.

The Rigor Wars

In the rigor wars, there are essentially two sides. One side insists that rigor must be maintained at all costs for the sake of education itself— this is the side of the rigor angsters. The other side insists that strict adherence to rigor for its own sake stands in the way of learning for all students, that is, inclusive teaching. The term "rigor wars" was coined by Professor Jamiella Brooks, who is the associate director of the Center for Teaching and Learning at the University of Pennsylvania.[4] Given how ugly some of the commentary has grown, "war" does not feel like an overstatement.

The argument that rigor and inclusive teaching cannot coexist was highlighted in a 2021 article by Professors Jordynn Jack and Viji Sathy ("It's Time to Cancel the Word 'Rigor'").[5] The authors rebut the notion that "abandoning 'rigorous' policies and assignments means lowering standards and watering down courses." Instead, they pull back the curtain on how the term "rigor" is most often used in higher education: as "code for 'some students deserve to be here, and some don't.'" Thus, rigor is a term of exclusion. Jack and Sathy focus on the exclusion of all marginalized students, so their critique of rigor is applicable to mentally disabled students. Recall that the opposite of exclusionary teaching is inclusion. Inclusion, in this context, means teaching accessibly, as Jack and Sathy model in their article.

Jack and Sathy show that what passes for rigor in most courses is simply a way of weeding out students. They explain: "Far too many faculty members still think a challenging course should be like an obstacle race: You, as the instructor, set up the tasks and each student has to finish them (or not) to a certain standard and within a set time. If only a few students can do it, that means the course is rigorous." In this way, the authors show how rigor angsters premise "rigor" on failure. This rigor/failure mindset leads to grading policies that allow for only a certain number of high grades, such as forced curves. The message these policies send to students is, as Jack and Sathy explain, "This instructor does not see all students as capable of success." But a forced curve is appealing to a teacher who fears their course might be perceived as unrigorous, because it ensures that some students will—by necessity—do poorly. Using a grading system that requires some students to do poorly or fail is a terrible stand-in for learning. Worse, though, such expectations of failure have a negative impact on student mental health.

Jack and Sathy insist that instead of focusing on weeding out students, faculty must focus on inclusive teaching: "Emphasize that students who have been admitted to your institution have already shown that they can meet high standards." Their point is that professors should believe that every student is capable of success, rather than starting the semester expecting some students to fail. As professors, it is our job to teach them to use their capabilities. In the context of mental disability, such inclusivity is at the heart of accessible teaching.

How does rigor angst exclude some students? Because, as Jack and Sathy explain, it "privilege[s] students who already have high academic literacy or who are already adept at managing higher education's unofficial rules, routines, and structures."[6] College, like every organization, has its unofficial rules and expectations. Many students arrive at college not knowing what those hidden rules and expectations are, even though they are well prepared for college-level coursework. These students include first-generation college students, students of color, nontraditional students, and more. These hidden rules are also ableist because they require students to decode social norms, skills that many mentally disabled students lack. Some mentally disabled students struggle with hidden rules even while they are well prepared academically.

Other scholars have supported Jack and Sathy's position, including Holden Thorp, chemistry professor and editor of the journal *Science*. In July of 2022, Thorp wrote an editorial ("Inclusion Doesn't Lower Standards") supporting inclusive pedagogy: "The rationale for this opposition [to inclusion] is often that 'accommodating' legitimate social and pedagogical needs of marginalized groups will lower the standards of mastery and excellence in these fields."[7] As Thorp points out, "this concern [over rigor] is just a crutch that protects faculty and institutions from having to do the work of correcting social injustices in higher education." Thorp's piece in such a lofty publication is a powerful response to myriad voices across the disciplines who cling to outdated notions about what it means to succeed in college and their fearmongering about lowering standards.

Rigor Angst in Action

Many professors have publicly defended "rigor," and close readings of these defenses reveal rigor angst. One such rigor angster, sociology professor Deborah J. Cohan, wrote a defense for *Inside Higher Ed* ("Upholding Rigor at Pandemic U"), that leads with this volley:

> If you've been following discussions on social media about pandemic pedagogy this past year, you've seen the conversations about how much to uphold pre-COVID standards of rigor and how much to cut students some slack. Virtually any post in which a faculty member sensitively conveys that they are stressed out about how much they can expect of students is met with what I would call the grace and compassion police, who insist faculty shouldn't demand very much from students. You know the type. They seem to be the same people who are the most performatively woke about anything and everything. [8]

In this passage, Cohan uses multiple strategies employed by those who want to attack others while avoiding criticism themselves. First is the word "police," which frames the writer as a victim. Cohan gives us a new type of "police" (not the "political correctness" police, for example); hers is the "grace and compassion police"—as though grace and compassion are bad things. Second, she uses the word "woke," a Black cultural term with a long civil-rights history dating back to the early twentieth century.[9] Over the last decade, "stay woke" and "woke" have referred to "always being on the lookout for systemic injustice"—except when appropriated by the people on the political right to criticize others for doing just those things. Teaching has really gotten toxic if professors are trying to spin grace, compassion, and righting systemic wrongs as bad things. Cohan's essay has not gotten off to a great start.

Cohan points to her twenty-six years of teaching experience, writing, "At a time when it is on trend to talk about ungrading, specs grading, labor-based grading and default grading of B and B-plus, it's hard to be the one person who's articulating that the full range of A through F grades may exist for a reason."[10] Cohan has a persecution complex—is she really the "one person" who wants to maintain a full grade scale? (Answer: no.) Is ungrading truly "on trend" in US higher education? (Answer: also no).

She criticizes professors who allow students to revise their work or turn it in late, by saying that they "lack boundaries." She compares these professors' actions to "self-sacrificial parenting," drawing a long comparison between students and children. It is not, therefore, surprising that she talks about her students as though they were children, which is, in itself, a problem because it infantilizes her adult students. With her words she also reveals that she views her students as children who are trying to trick her to get away with sneaky things, which is another, deeper problem, because it shows deep mistrust and even antagonism toward her students. She writes, "In the past year and a half, I've noticed a significant increase in the number of students who have emailed me vaguely claiming 'confusion' and 'stress' about anything and everything."[11] She does not believe her students when they tell her that they are struggling with their mental health. Instead, she is suspicious: "They've often also been the ones posting questions to their peers on social media about what the easiest classes are or where they can secure the gimme A's."[12] Thus, she concludes, "Confusion is frequently code for 'I haven't read the syllabus or the assignment.'"

Let's pause for a moment to do what Cohan has not done: listen to her students. They say that they are confused and stressed—indeed, about "anything and everything." Her students thus appear to be feeling an overwhelming, inchoate anxiety about life. It appears that this anxiety is spilling over into Cohan's class. My question is: Why is it so hard for Cohan to believe her students when they share their struggles with her? As I have shown frequently in this book, disclosing mental health struggles and asking professors for accommodations is hard. It is embarrassing, and students know that professors frequently meet these requests negatively.

Cohan says she does not believe her students because she has found her students on social media looking for easy As. Let's set aside my doubt that this professor is dogging her students' social media and grant that she found some posts by students looking for easier classes. But why did she allow those posts to erase all possibility that her students are also having mental health struggles? The two are not mutually exclusive. And honestly, if you were a student feeling exhausted and overwhelmed, might you reach out to friends to find a path to an easier A? Especially if you already understood that the cards were stacked against you by professors like Cohan?

When I began reading Cohan's piece, I did not expect to find it to be so silly and offensive. But every piece I have read defending rigor has been similarly silly and offensive. The problem is that the position is indefensible. Cohan has set up the pieces wrong: the rigor debate is not between pushover professors who lack boundaries and those who hold the line of excellence (like Cohan). That is a rigor war that exists only in Cohan's head. Good education and support of mental health struggles can, indeed, exist side by side. Supporting students is not coddling, and it need not lead to lower academic standards.

Other rigor angsters have written pieces that tread similar paths. For example, David Randall ("Don't Cancel Rigor") writes, regarding Jordynn Jack and Viji Sathy's piece: "Jack and Sathy's assault on rigor will remove the very ideal of excellence from our colleges."[13] Worse: "Jack and Sathy's pedagogical arguments are a stalking horse for differential standards by race and sex." Combine this language with Cohan's talk of "compassion police" and "woke" faculty, and you have a perfect right-wing conspiracy theory Mad Lib: woke faculty are using compassion to lower educational standards for people of color, women, and mentally stressed students. Or something like that.

Is It Really "Rigor"?

What I find most strange in the rigor angster essays is the lack of definition of the word. According to the *Oxford English Dictionary*, "rigor" (when not referring to death, i.e., rigor mortis) means a few things. It means "the quality of being extremely thorough, exhaustive, or accurate." It also means "severity or strictness." Looking at these two definitions, you can see that they do not mean the same thing: one refers to doing a good (thorough) job. One refers to being a jerk (severe, strict).

Do you have to be a jerk to get your students to do thorough work? Or can you be compassionate instead? As higher education journalist Beckie Supiano notes ("The Redefinition of Rigor"), the word "rigor" is meant to be used as "a synonym for 'challenging,' 'difficult,' or 'hard.'"[14] However, she points out, "some forms of challenge support learning; others are arbitrary obstacles that may well hinder it." How can you tell the difference?

If rigor is a synonym for "hard," then, I suggest, there can be "good-hard" and "bad-hard." Kevin Gannon, professor of history and director of the Teaching Center at Grand View University, helps explain the difference, "Courses can be difficult intellectually; they can be difficult logistically."[15] As Gannon explains, an intellectually difficult course "challenges students' assumptions, spurs their motivation, requires their effort, increases their skills." These courses "push students to learn." Thus, intellectual difficulty is good-hard. On the contrary, Gannon explains, "A logistically difficult course has strict policies about when and how work is produced and evaluated." Logistical difficulties are not about learning; they are obstacles to learning. They are bad-hard.

As Supiano points out, when professors reduce bad-hard work, they intend "to make students' lives easier, and probably it did."[16] However, this reduction in bad-hard work "does not necessarily mean students learned less or produced weaker work." In other words, courses remained good-hard. Gannon points out that COVID's stressors revealed the weaknesses in our old ways of thinking about course logistics.[17] "No single attendance policy can effectively deal with the complex health and personal situations" of our campus communities, no "single deadline policy" can account for students' obstacles to their learning, and "no lockstep approach to teaching modality" (i.e., only online or only in-person) can account for the health concerns of our community. Gannon emphasizes that the pandemic has taught us a "more humane approach to . . . teaching and learning," one with flexible logistics, and we should move forward with this new knowledge and put it to good use.

A similar point is made by Jamiella Brooks (the coiner of the term "rigor wars") and her colleague Julie McGurk (director of faculty teaching initiatives at Yale University's Poorvu Center for Teaching and Learning). In a presentation that has been highly influential in the rigor debate, they point out that they "do not think rigor is a bad teaching goal."[18] What they mean is that "having high standards for students communicates the professor's belief in their abilities, which helps students succeed. This is especially important, they note, for students categorized as members of minority groups." But they disagree with bad-hard teaching techniques that rigor angsters insist are rigorous. For example, grading on a forced bell curve, which only "compares students with their classmates but doesn't demonstrate what they know or learned."

Brooks and McGurk also criticize creating heavy assignments just for its own sake, noting that assigning a lot of work does not prove that a course is rigorous. Other experts have similarly weighed in on the quantity versus quality workload issue. Mays Imad, professor and coordinator of the Teaching and Learning Center at Pima Community College writes, "Establishing continuity doesn't mean you increase the amount of work required."[19]

When you take a big-picture look at all of the bad-hard teaching techniques espoused by rigor angsters, you will see how poisonous bad-hard coursework truly is. You will also see that what rigor angsters want is not about students' intellectual growth. Nurturing intellectual growth requires caring about your students on some level. At the very least, you are not cyberstalking them, being suspicious of them, or infantilizing them. No, what rigor angsters espouse is "toxic rigor," a term coined by faculty development professional and neurodiversity expert Karen Ray Costa in 2020.[20] I use "toxic rigor" to refer to the logistical rather than intellectual hurdles professors use in the classroom that infantilize students and reveal deep mistrust of them. (I delve deeper into toxic rigor in Chapter 11.)

Letting Go of Rigor Angst

Rigor angst is not new. The debate over forced grading curves and inclusive teaching was around long before COVID. The pandemic's stress has led to reshuffling of logistics and forced examination of curricula; this, in turn, has brought "rigor" to the forefront of higher education policy once again. But this new debate over rigor can lead to good changes in teaching and policy if we allow it.

Pandemic rigor angst arose when faculty had to move their courses online suddenly. Most of these professors were not online educators, and they feared that rigor would slip because of the distance-learning format: students would fail to pay attention; they would not take school seriously; they would goof off during online class (more so, I suppose, than they did during in-person class).

In the context of online learning, rigor angst arose from what Dr. Lee Skallerup Bessette, a learning design specialist at Georgetown University, calls a "deficit mentality" about online teaching.[21] This deficit mentality arises when a person envisions online teaching only as a poor substitute for in-person teaching. Designing an online course is not the same thing as scrambling to keep the semester alive. Skallerup Bessette urged professors to keep an open mind: "Online pedagogy does offer a form of intimacy and intensity," even if it is different from in-person teaching.[22] Online education has its own benefits to offer our students, different benefits from in-person learning. Faculty need to adjust our mindsets and be willing to figure out what those benefits are, especially as it appears that online learning, in some form, is here to stay (and that's a good thing).

I am with Gannon: intellectual challenges are what matter. Logistical landmines do not. I am also with Brooks and McGurk when they say that burying students in content does not make students learn more. In fact, one of the first changes I made after COVID hit was to cut back the number of individual writing assignments my students had to complete in my advanced legal writing course. Instead, I had my students do more peer review and revision of a smaller number of writing assignments. My mantra was "go deeper, not wider." I discovered that the course was better for the change. A 2022 study later supported my choice to cut the breadth of content and use active learning methods to engage more deeply with the material.[23] After publishing the findings, the lead author on the study wrote on social media, "Let's be brave and reduce content."[24] I kept the new course design after we returned to in-person teaching. My takeaway from the pandemic was an examination of my course to discover which assignments were difficult just for the sake of being difficult, and a transformation of those assignments into ones that generated actual intellectual challenge—and learning.

I encourage you to strip away your habitual notions of rigor, as I did. Look for what is bad-hard versus good-hard; look for what is toxic. Let's lighten (or scrap) as much bad-hard work as we can. Review your syllabus and its course requirements. Do you have logistical difficulties that you can make easier? Do so. Your students will learn more because they are worrying less about logistics. Then ask yourself, *What course structure will foster the deepest learning by the greatest number of students?* Come up with a list of principles based on the answers to that question, then design your course around those principles.

11

Toxic Rigor Is Ableist

When I was a young professor teaching freshman composition, I took attendance. I thought I was supposed to in order to encourage students to come to class. However, I thought that I was wonderfully forward thinking because I gave my students three free absences during the semester. In fact, I was so forward thinking that they did not even have to give me an excuse: "Just give me a heads up that you won't be coming. I don't need you to give me a reason," I would say to them at the beginning of each semester. "Email me, *Dear Professor Pryal, I apologize, but I won't be able to attend class today*. I don't want to hear about your vomit or whatever." The vomit joke always got a bunch of laughs. And you know what? My students thought my attendance policy was awesome. Even though after three absences I started docking their final grades.

In the spring semester of 2009 when I gave this talk to my students at UNC–Chapel Hill, I added something like this at the end of the speech: "So, look. This semester you might want to hang onto these free absences. We have a habit of winning national basketball championships." We had a very good men's basketball team that year, and my freshmen might not have known just how good we were. And indeed we won, and the day after, I got many emails that said:

> Dear Professor Pryal, I apologize, but I won't be able to attend class today. WOOOHOOO.

Or some variation. And when I received each one, I laughed. Only seven students came to class, and I didn't mind at all.

After a student used up their three absences, though, I started taking points off their final grades. No excuses. Even if a student turned in perfect work all semester, enough to earn an A, if they missed four class meetings, the highest grade they could earn was an A-. If they missed five, the highest grade they could earn was a B+. Some students begged me to make exceptions, but I held firm. I thought I was teaching them responsibility. (Spoiler alert: I was not.)

Eventually I ended up teaching in a law school, where the American Bar Association requires a student to attend 80 percent of class meetings in order to avoid an automatic incomplete. I put the ABA rule on my syllabus as required by the law school. When I started, I thought that it was a good rule because it taught law students professionalism. In retrospect, I also liked the rule because it took the job of managing attendance out of my hands—no more pleading from students. When a student got close to missing 20 percent of the course, I would let them know. They would give me a scared look and dash off. My job was done. And if they missed more classes? Well, that was out of my hands.

But I was wrong, so wrong, about the lessons my students learned from these strict attendance policies. I thought I was doing the right thing. Teaching responsibility and professionalism. Teaching students to plan ahead. Instead, I taught students that no matter what crises life throws at them—illness, death, harm, mental health struggles—no one will care, and they don't deserve sympathy or respect.

I was also wrong that what counted as an absence was so black and white. Despite being a contingent faculty member and later an adjunct, a professor with the least amount of power at just about any institution, I still had vast control over my courses. I could have determined what counted as an excused absence. I could have determined what make-up work could turn an unexcused absence into an excused one. I had the power to help my students succeed; I just chose not to use it.

Literally everything I thought I knew about attendance was incorrect. Worse, it was ableist pedagogy. When I look back on what I did, what I believed, I cringe. I have to forgive my former self. More importantly, I have to ask forgiveness of my former students. Now I have to make up for what I did wrong in the past by helping all of us understand more about how ableist pedagogies have snuck into our mindsets and taken hold without our realizing it. Let's take a conscious look at the ableist pedagogical choices that we make, instead of defaulting to the norm.

Here we go.

What Is Toxic Rigor?

As a result of the COVID pandemic, the long-running "rigor wars" in higher education have come to the fore.[1] On one side, you have those who believe that good education and support of mental health struggles (or any student struggles) can exist side by side. On the other you have those who believe that support of students is coddling, and coddling waters down academic standards—that is, rigor. What this second group of professors feel is what I call "rigor angst," the fear that a curriculum will not be difficult enough to meet certain academic standards. Rigor angsters assuage their fears with "toxic rigor,"[2] logistical hurdles that infantilize students and reveal deep mistrust of them. Examples include punitive mandatory attendance policies, strict deadlines with few exceptions for extensions, required in-person instruction even for those with disabilities or illnesses who would be safer learning online, refusing to post class recordings or lecture notes online unless forced to by disability services, not allowing laptops in class (again, unless forced to), and more. (I delve deeply into rigor angst, the rigor wars, and toxic rigor in Chapter 10, "Rigor Angst.")

Toxic rigor is deeply ableist because rigor angst is a manifestation of ableism. Rigor angsters see accommodating a disabled student as giving that student "a leg up." They're suspicious of students asking for accommodations: "Honestly, how does every kid have a diagnosis these days? They're faking ADHD to get extra time on tests." Rigor angsters believe accessible teaching is teaching to the "lowest common denominator." They are unable to see that learning accommodations create a level playing field, allowing a disabled student to have an equal chance at learning. Instead, they fear that disability accommodations will "water down" their courses—that is, make them less rigorous.

The "Disability Con"

It is not a stretch to say that when rigor angsters perceive that academic standards are loosened, they freak out with fear that our education system is going to fall to pieces. In 2021, one rigor angster wrote that, if we lose rigor, it "will cripple American higher education."[3] This professor used the word "cripple," an ableist metaphor. The rest of his rigor argument is transparently ableist.

For example, he rejects "getting rid of grading on a curve, as well as adopting frequent low-stakes tests" and also "'group learning,' that banality the education schools have been foisting up and down the education system."[4] Grading on a curve ensures that some students will, by necessity, do poorly in a class. These students who do poorly are stand-ins for rigor—after all, if everyone does well, a professor's course cannot have been rigorous, right? Wrong—that course is toxic, sacrificing some students' success to appease the professor's need to appear tough. Curves are toxic because they express the expectation, at the beginning of a semester, that some students will do poorly, which has a negative impact on students' mental health and their desire to study at all. Decades-old research shows that curves decrease student motivation. A 2009 study showed that "absolute grading is better than grading on a curve" when it comes to creating student incentives to study.[5] A course that has only a few high-stakes exams (or, in the case of law school, only *one*), each graded on a curve, creates intense pressure on mentally disabled students. Alternatively, having multiple low-stakes tests, each graded accurately (called "absolute grading"), decreases test anxiety and shows faith in students' ability to succeed.

Accommodations are another front of the rigor wars. Many faculty, not just rigor angsters, use the term "accommodations" to refer to adjustments to curriculum, even though they are not, at least outwardly, referring to disability. I do not believe it is coincidental that the word "accommodations" has been used to describe the learning adjustments faculty have made (or refused to make) due to student struggles, whether mental health related or not. Widespread mental disability accommodations have long been a battleground of the rigor wars, whether rigor angsters use the D-word or not.

In US disability law, "accommodations" connotes something extra that is given to a disabled person. And, the reasoning goes, because accommodations are extra, they can and should be taken away when they are no longer needed. But who makes that decision? In the context of the pandemic, when 2021 rolled around, rigor angsters started calling for the extra pandemic accommodations to be dropped in favor of a return to (toxic) rigor. They argued that we were harming our students because we were treating them as "too mentally ill or too traumatized to function."[6] Beneath rigor angsters' call for a "return" to academic standards was the belief that supporting student mental health and providing a good education cannot possibly coexist.

But rigor angst is not just a fear of academic standards dropping; it is the fear of *why*. It is the suspicion of students, the us-versus-them mentality that rigor angsters show in their arguments about rigor. It is the fear that our students are faking being traumatized or mentally disabled so that they can slack off or get easy As.[7] This suspicion of disabled people faking their disabilities is embedded in our culture. In the United States more broadly and higher education specifically, there is a "cultural anxiety" that some people will "fake disabilities to take advantage of rights, accommodations, or benefits."[8] This anxiety about disability fakery is what disability legal studies scholar Doron Dorfman calls the "fear of the disability con."[9] Dorfman shows that, in popular discourse, arguments proliferate that disabled people "gain an unfair advantage by 'disguising' their demands as striving to achieve 'equal rights' and an 'even playing field' when they are actually seeking 'extra benefits.'" This concern about fakery, the disability con, causes suspicion of disabled people. As a result of this widespread suspicion, our institutions put in place policies that require disabled students (and faculty) to go to great and unnecessary lengths to prove that they are disabled in order to gain needed accommodations. This "accommodation discrimination," as disability legal studies scholar Katherine A. Macfarlane puts it, results in many disabled students being unable to gain accommodations at all.[10]

Accommodations Cost Too Much

What is ironic is that disability accommodations are extremely difficult to acquire, despite the rigor angster narrative to the contrary. Put simply, accommodations cost too much: too much money, too much time, and too much emotional strain. For example, students who seek accommodations for their mental disabilities must pay for expensive neurological, educational, and psychological testing. They must find a doctor who will perform the tests and transportation to get to the doctor. They must find the time to take the tests. Macfarlane notes that schools require new medical documentation far too frequently—some require new testing every three years. Each time, a student must pay for an evaluation that costs hundreds to thousands of dollars.[11] Furthermore, as Macfarlane shows, these policies have a disproportionate negative impact on students who are racial minorities. Our society's suspicion of disability fakery creates a society-wide acceptance of this high standard of proof that disabled students (and all disabled people) must show in order to have necessary accommodations of their disabilities—proof that is not required by federal law.

Suspicion of disability fakery has many other negative effects for disabled people, including resentment by abled people, as Dorfman's research reveals: "The desirability of [disability] accommodations by nondisabled people evokes jealousy and allows these rights to be recast as 'special treatment.'"[12] Jealousy creates the popular belief that special treatment is "prone to fakery and abuse." For example, in a classroom where a rigor angster bans laptops, a disabled person who is allowed to use one because of a disability accommodation will be subject to the jealousy and resentment of their classmates who are not allowed to use them. Furthermore, the disabled student will be "outed" as disabled because of their laptop use. The solution is simple: don't ban laptops; it is ableist and toxic pedagogy reflecting only a mistrust of students.[13]

The fear of the disability con also negatively affects the mental health of disabled people. Dorfman's quantitative research shows that nearly 60 percent of disabled Americans believe that others question their disability.[14] Respondents shared how this ongoing suspicion negatively affects their lives. One disabled respondent wrote: "Because there is no outward evidence of my problem, I have to explain it for someone to know about it. I have had to tell hundreds, maybe thousands of people about my personal medical problem over the last 22 years."[15] The suspicion of fakery Dorfman describes is yet another aspect of ableism that disabled people have to deal with.

In higher education, the fear of the disability con is rampant. As disability studies scholar Jay T. Dolmage writes, disabled students "are already routinely and systematically constructed as faking it, jumping a queue, or asking for an advantage."[16] In particular, Dolmage points out, "so-called invisible disabilities" face even greater suspicion. As I noted in the introduction to this book, mental disabilities are frequently "invisible," often because the disabled person works hard to hide them. For example, autistic students often mask their autism; other neurodivergent students take similar steps to appear neurotypical. Students do this exhausting work of hiding their disabilities because of fear of stigma. At the same time, their disabled status is questioned because they appear "normal." Thus, mentally disabled students face a double bind: if you appear too disabled, you are ostracized. If you mask your disability, you don't deserve accommodations.

Under the accommodations model, there will always be disabled students jumping through hoops to get services or exceptions, and there will always be gatekeepers (administrators, professors) blocking their way. Mere accommodation of disabilities is not enough; we must teach accessibly instead. As I've written extensively in this book, accommodations are not accessibility. Margaret Price draws the distinction between accommodation and accessibility in higher education like this: "Accommodation, while helpful, is often used to indicate specific measures intended to 'fix' specific situations for individual 'problems.' Access means designing spaces . . . in ways that are flexible, multi-modal, and responsive to feedback."[17] Accessible spaces are always, all the time, welcoming to all disabled students, "no hoops required" for them to jump through.[18]

Mismanaged Accommodations

Rigor angst has long haunted campus disability accommodations. Students have to worry about rigor angst any time they request course accommodations from their institutions, including from faculty. In a 2017 article in the *Chronicle of Higher Education* ("Why I Dread the Accommodations Talk"), psychology professor Gail A. Hornstein describes how she (mis)handles student accommodation requests for mental disabilities.[19] She tells a story of meeting with a student, during which the student shared her medical diagnosis of panic disorder to defend her need for accommodations. The student was afraid she might have an attack during an exam, for example. (A student should never, ever have to share their private medical information with a professor. In fact, it's illegal to pressure them to do so.) Then Hornstein took it upon herself to give the student guidance that is beyond her training:

> I relaxed into my chair, and looked directly at Lee. "Well, I hope that doesn't happen," I said evenly. "This course has a very fast pace, each assignment builds on the ones prior, and you'd be at a significant disadvantage if you missed a test. You're a psych major,

and this is our most important course. I know you want to do well in it. Let's talk about how to make sure that happens."

Hornstein wrote with odd pride that Lee "never again came to my office"—as though Lee avoided her because she no longer needed her, and couldn't possibly be avoiding her because the professor made her uncomfortable. Then she writes, wrongly yet again, these words: "Students certainly have needs, but those often have little to do with what's on their accommodation forms," disparaging the hard work that disability services offices do to prepare those accommodation forms in the first place.

Finally, for our purposes, she shows how poorly she understands mental disabilities, and disabilities generally: "Compared with physical disabilities, psychiatric conditions are far more variable—both for different people with the same diagnosis and even for the same person at different times or in different contexts."[20] (Recall that she is a professor of psychology.) Her words are wrong for a number of reasons: physical disabilities are just as variable as mental disabilities, for example, and to treat them as monolithic discriminates against all disabled people whose physical abilities vary from day to day or week to week. She continues, describing mental disabilities: "People aren't equally anxious, depressed, dissociated, subject to panic attacks, or even learning disabled all the time, or necessarily in all the same ways." Well, obviously; all disabilities are variable depending on many factors. But she uses the variability of mental disabilities to argue that mentally disabled people do not deserve the same degree of accommodation as physically disabled people.

Based on this faulty premise, the author then advises faculty to overstep their jobs—and violate the law—rather than provide the institution-approved accommodations to mentally disabled students. She urges faculty to "help students to learn what's a crisis (and what's not), and to understand when it is reasonable to ask for the course structure to be changed or for expectations to be modified (and when it's best to try to cope on one's own)." She thus encourages students to see that sometimes their accommodations are not "reasonable"—even when their own institution judges that they are, even when the student thinks that they are. When accommodations are unreasonable, students must "cope on [their] own" rather than expect disability accommodations.

But who decides what is unreasonable? The professor, of course. She speaks of teaching disabled students how to understand what is unreasonable. But what she is actually teaching is that their professor is ableist (if we're lucky) or to internalize ableism (if we're unlucky). Disabled students walk away from her course either hating their professor or hating themselves.

Furthermore, she is encouraging all professors to ignore students' legally binding accommodation requests. Why? Her explanation: "We aren't helping students who already have problems to succeed in their lives after college by treating them in a standardized manner or by over-protecting them." In other words, she believes accommodations are "overprotective"—another way of saying that they are a leg up rather than creating a level playing field. Then, instead of granting a student's accommodations, she urges professors to determine what *lesser* accommodations are needed, a task that they are not suited for nor legally able to do: "Determining who actually requires assistance, and in what form, and discouraging students from defining themselves by what they can't do can be especially important." Thus, she writes, faculty must figure out which students "actually" need accommodations so that students who have "problems" are not "overprotected" or taught to "define themselves" by their disabilities. The language that students should not "define themselves" by their disabilities implies that students are ashamed of their disabilities. But the only shaming happening here is perpetrated by professors disregarding accommodations.

Despite its cruelty, Hornstein's essay provides a useful look inside the brain of an accommodations gatekeeper, revealing that her refusal to grant accommodations is driven by toxic rigor. She writes, "Of course we must take their individual needs into account and make sensible accommodations when warranted."[21] With these words, Hornstein implies that it is her job to determine what is sensible. This is such a dangerous argument because she believes she—and the faculty readers of her column—understand accommodations better than their disabled students and the disability services office. The reason for her advice? Rigor. It is "our responsibility as faculty members to uphold educational standards, to ensure fairness, and to model resourcefulness for all students, no matter their background or life challenges." The phrase "uphold educational standards" reveals the author's rigor angst; when she pairs it with "ensure fairness," a catchphrase that reveals fear of disability fakery, she reveals how inextricable rigor angst and ableism truly are. For rigor angsters, toxic rigor and disability accommodations cannot coexist.

What Do We Do?

Through professional training, we must separate intellectual rigor from toxicity and angst. Professors must learn what it means to teach accessibly instead of with fear of disability fakery. If they can do so, they can create an environment driven not by fear but by collaboration between professor and students. The relationships between students and professors need not be adversarial.

I believe rigor can, indeed, mean deep, intellectual work (as it did before rigor angsters turned it toxic). And this kind of work can easily coexist with accessible teaching. Accessibility can become the norm if an institution puts its will behind creating an environment that is welcoming and inclusive of disabled students. I also believe that most professors want to do the right thing. They just don't understand that toxic rigor is the enemy of the right thing—or even that some of their policies reflect toxic rigor at all.

The pandemic has made so many things confusing, but it has also made many things clearer. As I have pointed out more than once in this book, mental disability and mental health struggles have long been a crisis in higher education. It only took a pandemic to bring them into the light.

We must refuse to let them be shoved into the dark again. Instead, we must teach with a pedagogy focused on student learning instead of toxic, meaningless metrics—such as a forced curve, which "arbitrarily limits the number of students who can excel."[22] At the same time, our pedagogy must also focus on our students surviving with their spirits intact—and, in some cases, surviving, period. We must allow our students to make mistakes without punitive consequences. Instead, we must teach students how failures can and should be learning experiences—*that* is how you teach resilience.[23] We can change our schema of assignments so that our students' grades do not depend only on one or two large tasks—and thereby depressurize the semester. We can rethink deadlines; at the same time, we can teach students how to ask for extensions, an important life skill.[24]

I believe that if any student fails my class, I have failed as a professor. A professor's job is to make sure that every student learns the curriculum so that they can move forward in their education. Our students do not need toxic conditions in order to learn, and we as professors do not need these conditions to assuage our fears that we are not teaching well. Instead, build relationships with your students and have faith in yourself, and in them.

12

Teaching Mentally Disabled Students

I recently met Emma, an autistic student at a mid-Atlantic university, who shared with me some of her experiences as a mentally disabled student in college. She described how "a professor can make or break your experience" in a course. For Emma, the best professors "made me feel like I belonged in the class," as opposed to other professors who only "followed through with my accommodations because they were legally obligated." Mentally disabled students like Emma can tell which professors care about their success and which professors don't. They can also tell which professors see them as a burden and which genuinely welcome them into their classrooms.

We should want to be professors who welcome mentally disabled (i.e., neurodivergent) students. As a practical matter, they make up a large number of our students. More importantly, however, rather than being a burden, they have much to offer our classrooms. Our job is not *only* to grant the accommodations that students bring us from disability services, as Emma described, but also to create an accessible space where all disabled students can learn, whether they are officially recognized by disability services or not. "Accommodations" are special exceptions for one person and require lots of work on the part of the disabled person to acquire. "Accessibility" means creating a space that is welcoming to and usable by disabled people. It doesn't require disabled people to do extra work the way accommodations do.

(Another way to think about accessible teaching is Universal Design for Learning, which is "a teaching approach that works to accommodate the needs and abilities of all learners and eliminates unnecessary hurdles in the learning process.")[1]

An accessible approach for teaching mentally disabled students gains even more importance when you remember that mentally disabled students are not monolithic. Their needs vary, even among those with the same diagnosis. The accommodations model fails because it provides a one-size-fits-all response to ADHD, autism, anxiety, and so forth: a quiet room for exams, extra time—necessary accommodations for sure, but not enough. The accessibility model creates a learning environment where students can, ideally, have access to any of the learning tools they need to succeed.

Mentally Disabled Students in Our Classrooms

As faculty, we can't know how many mentally disabled students are in our courses. We also can't know what academic advisers and disability services are doing for our mentally disabled students. Finally, we can't know whether our mentally disabled students are receiving help from these outside resources at all.

There is one thing we can know for sure: we have many mentally disabled students in our classrooms. Up to 2 percent of college students are autistic.[2] Students with ADHD make up 19 percent of college students.[3] Many more have anxiety disorders and depression.[4] Many of these mental disabilities make it difficult to process information, organize and prioritize tasks, and more.[5] None of these difficulties say anything about these students' intellectual abilities—only about how much harder college can be for them than it is for neurotypical students.

Keep in mind, though, that mentally disabled students are hardly a monolith. Faculty development professional and neurodiversity expert Karen Ray Costa, who has ADHD, explained to me in an interview, "Know that even within specific ND [neurodivergent] groups, there is a lot of variation." So what should professors do? Costa told me, "Use your intersectional and relational lens to design and teach." To do so, professors should form relationships with our students. As Costa put it: "In short, get to know your learners."

One way you can get to know your students is to use an anonymous survey at the beginning of the semester. Give this survey to everyone in your class, asking them to identify tactics that will help them learn. You will need to provide some examples to help them understand the question and the scope of the possible answers. Encourage creativity.

You can't know what diversity of challenges your students are facing. You may have students who are full-time parents, for example, who are therefore getting little sleep or struggling with postpartum illness. These students (and others) have needs that do not fall squarely into the box of disability, but nevertheless create mental health struggles that need to be accounted for. A survey will help you get to know your students better and therefore help you teach better.

It is also important to avoid stereotyping mental disabilities. For instance, autism is a spectrum, and every autistic student is unique. As autistic professor Maggie Coughlin points out, "If you know one person on the spectrum, you know one person on the spectrum."[6] Stereotyping leads to stigma, pushing the lived reality of autistic students to the shadows. Stereotyping can occur in class discussions, for example. In clinical research, autistic students have reported "experiencing stigmatizing classroom discussions on autism that did not recognize that some students in the room may identify as autistic."[7]

Similarly, every ADHD student has unique strengths and challenges. ADHD is stereotypically seen as a total lack of ability to focus. This stereotype ignores ADHD "hyperfocus," the ability some people with ADHD have to "concentrate intently for long stretches of time on complex projects."[8] If students with ADHD are able to explore meaningful work or if they have the right situational supports to enable them to do so, they have a strong ability to focus on their work.

ADHD students face another insidious stereotype: the disability faker who is trying to game the system.[9] There is an all-too-common myth that ADHD diagnoses are widely abused to help students cheat.[10] This awful stereotype stigmatizes students who have a serious disability.

Despite the high number of mentally disabled students in your classroom, you might not get many students who disclose their disabled status to you. Why not? First, getting accommodations in college is a struggle, and many fail to get them. Law professor and disability expert Kat Macfarlane recounts the hurdles disabled students face:

> All new college students experience stress, but disabled students experience additional stress because they must deal with seeking accommodations in addition to learning how to be a college student.

Disabled students must provide invasive and expensive medical documentation to prove they are disabled.

Many disabled students on campus will have lost the support systems that they had at home that provided additional support for their disabilities and seeking accommodations.

Students must do extensive self-advocacy with disability services offices and their professors, creating yet another barrier.[11]

Students also must face the challenge of disability services offices who do not have enough staff to serve all students—a top-level administrative failure. Research findings show that disabled students experience "disability service offices [that] are understaffed and can therefore assist only those students with the most urgent needs."[12]

Next, there are those students like I was, who might be unaware that they are mentally disabled at all. I was diagnosed with bipolar disorder in my twenties, and then, twenty years later, with autism. Thus, I spent all of my college years with serious mental disabilities and no diagnoses. Later, I spent my graduate school years with no diagnosis of autism because, like 80 percent of autistic women, I didn't receive a diagnosis in childhood.[13] Indeed, in a foundational study that sought to discover the prevalence of autism among college students, *every* student whom the researchers screened positive for autism had never been diagnosed before.[14] Those researchers and other well-respected organizations now recommend that colleges start screening students for autism because it is so underdiagnosed.[15]

Finally, many mentally disabled students keep their accommodation needs to themselves because they fear the stigma against mental disability. Stigma means "shame," and in higher education, any mental disability is—still—considered shameful. After all, higher education is about learning, which is about brains—and if your brain isn't perfect, what does that say about you? Stigma against mental disability is one manifestation of ableism.

Stigma can manifest as the internalized belief held by a disabled student that they don't really need or deserve accommodations. Eric Garcia, autistic journalist and author of *We're Not Broken: Changing the Autism Conversation*, describes how, after he enrolled in college, he "felt that if I used special accommodations. . . . I was somehow cheating."[16] He writes, "I feared I would be taking a shortcut if I got help that

I felt I didn't 'really need.'" Garcia, like many mentally disabled students, had internalized the ableism that many in higher education feel toward mentally disabled students who seek accommodations: that accommodations are an unfair leg up or cheating, and therefore something to be ashamed of.

Because being disabled and asking for accommodations can be a source of embarrassment, even students who are registered with disability services might choose to hide their status from professors. Some students have been humiliated by professors in the past and therefore choose to avoid disclosing to professors again in the future, even if doing so puts their education at risk. (In Chapter 11, "Toxic Rigor is Ableist," I recount the story of a professor who refused to honor a mentally disabled student's accommodations for her panic disorder, instead insisting that she muscle through the course.)

My student friend Emma told me a story about a professor who refused to follow the accommodations from her institution's disability services center. Emma was supposed to be allowed to take the exams in the university's proctoring center, a location designed for disabled students to take exams. Instead, Emma told me, "He made me take them in a secluded room in the building the class was in," disregarding an important aspect of her accommodations. To be clear: disregarding a student's accommodations is illegal. It is also unethical and cruel. Don't do it.

Many professors feel uncomfortable when students approach them to ask for accommodations. If you feel that way, that's okay. Because of the stigma against mental disabilities, discussing disabilities can feel taboo, but it doesn't need to. When a student discloses to you, they probably feel uncomfortable too. They may expect you to feel annoyed that you have to accommodate them or, worse, doubtful that their disabilities are real.

If a student does you the honor of disclosing their disability to you, strive to be open-minded and empathetic. You might find such conversations awkward, so here is some welcoming language:

> Thank you for sharing your disability with me. I appreciate the trust you have put in me. Your educational success is important to me, so I would like to make this class as accessible as possible for you. What are the accommodations that you will find most helpful?

After the student tells you those accommodations, grant them.

We must all recognize how difficult it is for our mentally disabled students to get accommodations through our institutions. Recognize that accommodations are not actually handed out like candy and instead reflect a true need. And also recognize that we have students who need accommodations but do not have institutional recognition because of very real roadblocks—yet they still need our help. Here are some ideas for how to teach accessibly for those students who don't have official accommodations.

Scaffold Assignments to Aid Executive Function

In the educational context, scaffolding means to provide interim structure to larger assignments. Research has shown that autistic students benefit from scaffolded assignments, which "can lower the anxiety of students with ASD and play to their strengths of thriving in structured environments."[17] Furthermore, scaffolding benefits mentally disabled students because they frequently struggle with "executive function." Executive function refers to the mental skills that all people need to accomplish our goals. Executive function challenges can cause problems with starting and finishing tasks, completing multistep tasks, staying on track with big projects, planning and organizing projects, and balancing multiple responsibilities.[18] Executive function struggles are common in students with autism, ADHD, anxiety disorders, and depression. Thus, scaffolding benefits the large number of students in your classes who are mentally disabled.

Here is an example of how to implement scaffolding. You can scaffold a large writing assignment, such as a final seminar paper, by breaking the assignment into smaller tasks. To reduce the load on you—we faculty do *not* need to increase our workloads—do not evaluate each of these smaller assignments. For example, you can simply review them in your course management software to make sure no one is falling behind.

Here are some suggestions for smaller assignments: have each student write a brief proposal for their paper, then an annotated bibliography, then an outline. They can give peer feedback on any or all of these assignments with a cohort from class. If you choose to do peer feedback, be sure to provide instruction for how to do so. Peer feedback is not something that comes naturally to our students, especially to mentally disabled students, for whom social interactions can be fraught. Providing a framework for peer feedback can be a big relief for mentally disabled students—and *all* students. Scaffolding a large assignment should also reduce your grading work because the seminar papers your students turn in will likely be of higher quality—and you'll get fewer papers that are far off track.

You can also scaffold reading assignments. If you assign readings to learn your course content—say, from a biology textbook, it is likely you already know what you want your students to get out of each day's reading. Instead of sending them on a reading treasure hunt to discover the important points, provide guidance before they start. This guidance is critical for many mentally disabled readers, for whom it can be difficult to discern what is important in assigned reading. For some mentally disabled readers, the part of the reading they find fascinating might not be important at all to the learning goals. Reading for classes becomes a puzzle to decipher rather than a tool for learning. Consider this: the purpose of reading a biology textbook is to learn biology. It is not to decipher complex ideas from a text. Thus, you shouldn't expect your students to do that kind of work. (Of course, some courses *do* expect readers to do that work—literature classes for example.)

In their book *Inclusive Teaching: Strategies for Promoting Equity in the College Classroom*, Kelly A. Hogan and Viji Sathy note that "some students will feel overwhelmed and lost if a large amount of reading is assigned."[19] You can scaffold a reading assignment by providing a list of key ideas that you want students to take away from it. Such a list helps students read with a purpose rather than trying to puzzle out the important parts or going down rabbit holes. To make this key ideas list without adding much to your workload, use the ideas you already have planned for discussion. You might be thinking that giving your students a list of key ideas for their reading is hand-holding—but it isn't. Instead, we are preventing our students from feeling anxious because the reading didn't teach them anything but to try to read our minds. A key ideas list ensures that our students learn the material instead.

Finally, you can scaffold your lectures and class discussions. For many mentally disabled students, determining what is important in a lecture or class discussion can be difficult, no matter how powerful their intellect. This is because many mentally disabled students struggle with working memory, which is the brain's ability to quickly process unfamiliar information.[20] (Working memory is a component of executive function.)

How can you ensure that all of your students are learning from your class lectures and discussions? When you are planning your lectures or class discussions, provide in advance what Hogan and Sathy call "skeletal outlines."[21] These outlines will help mentally disabled students, and *any* students, who might become overwhelmed by all of the information in a lecture. Hogan and Sathy explain that these outlines provide a document that "students can take notes on, so that they don't have to write everything down, but must stay actively engaged to fill in *parts* of the outline."[22] These outlines help students organize and prioritize information.

We can prepare these outlines with minimal labor. As we plan class, we plan what we will cover each week. If you have not been much of a planner in the past, know that this planning will make you a better teacher—it has for me. It makes you think hard about what is necessary to include in class and how to best organize it. When you write lecture or discussion notes, reduce those notes into a skeletal outline and give them to your students. Do not worry if you don't stick closely to your plan. Like many professors, I, too, sometimes wing it during class discussions. That's fine. Giving our students an outline is better than giving them nothing at all.

Reframing Paying Attention

When I was in graduate school, like many of my classmates, I wrote about my ideas in a composition book. During class, unlike my classmates, I wrote about *lots* of ideas in those notebooks. In fact, I wrote *nonstop*—taking notes from discussion and processing the ideas that flowed during class. As time went on, my incessant writing led some of my professors to assume that I was off task, ignoring class and noodling around in my notebook about something unrelated.

One particular professor tried more than once to "catch" me not paying attention by cold-calling on me during discussion: "And what do YOU think, Katie?" Because I was, indeed, paying attention, I cheerfully answered the questions. At first, I was oblivious to the accusatory tone, because that's what can happen when you're autistic. Eventually, I did catch on to the mean-spiritedness. And when I did, my feelings were deeply hurt. Why didn't the professor just talk to me instead of trying to publicly humiliate me?

Karen Ray Costa told me that mentally disabled student behavior (like mine) is frequently misunderstood by professors. As Costa explains, when a student is doodling or, say, scribbling endlessly like I did, professors sometimes think poorly about the student. She told me that professors assume that a "student isn't paying attention because that's not the model that they hold of what attention looks like. But," Costa explained, "attention is nuanced and complex." Put more simply, given the presence of mentally disabled students in our courses, we, as faculty, need to rethink our notions of what it means to be a well-behaved student.

Some mentally disabled students find it stressful to maintain eye contact. They also find it easier to process information by looking away from the slide deck, professor, or whiteboard. This looking away is called "gaze aversion." As one disability advocacy group explains about autistic people in particular, "Gaze aversion is a sensory processing tool, one necessary to managing sensory overwhelm."[23] Furthermore, "when an autistic person looks away, we are thinking and processing. We *are* paying attention. There is a lot of processing and parsing going on within."[24] In fact, clinical research shows that gaze aversion is important to processing for *all* people.[25]

Sometimes it might appear that a mentally disabled student isn't paying attention when actually they're focused inward, trying to process all of the information coming their way. These mini "brain breaks" allow some mentally disabled students to concentrate on what they've just heard and turn it into knowledge. (I did this same processing work by writing in my grad school notebook, transforming the class ideas into my own.) As Costa explained to me, "Often, neurotypical professors (and sometimes ND [neurodivergent] professors too) have a belief system about what 'paying attention' looks like." And if a student doesn't line up with that belief system, the student isn't paying attention properly in class. Our job as faculty is to rethink what paying attention looks like and shake off the normate stereotype, allowing room for neurodiversity in our classrooms. The stereotype of a student "spacing out" in class is just that—a stereotype. Let us set it aside and allow students to engage how they see fit.

On a similar note, we can rethink how class discussions look. Many mentally disabled students want to participate in discussion, but the way many discussions are structured excludes them. This exclusion can also be attributed to working memory challenges—for those of us who struggle with working memory, when information is flying at us during a discussion, it can take us a moment to put that information in an order that makes sense. In certain circumstances, when we are familiar with the information's context, we can do fine. But if we are not familiar, we need some time.

As faculty, during a class discussion, it is tempting to call on the first student who raises their hand. I know I've done that. But instead, consider that someone who is mentally disabled might raise their hand *last*, after processing all of the new information that has been presented. Consider alternating between the early hand-raisers and the late ones. It's okay to let hands hang in the air for a bit. When you do so, you might find you have new and exciting contributions from students you haven't heard from before.

Accessible Course Design

Emma, the autistic student I interviewed, told me she feared her professors would judge her if they knew she was autistic. She was particularly afraid in her dance class. "In the beginning," Emma told me, "I kept my neurodivergence a secret from my dance professors." She told me why: "I didn't want my professors to think that I wasn't capable of performing because of my neurodivergence." However, later in the semester, Emma made a choice to share: "I eventually did tell them because, ultimately, autism is part of my identity and sometimes I do need accommodations." Emma's story led me to ask: How can we design our courses so that mentally disabled students know, from the get-go, that they can succeed in our classes?

Research shows that professors' attitudes toward their students' learning disabilities make a big difference in students' success.[26] One study showed that students performed better in classrooms where professors were "receptive when they disclosed their [learning] disability."[27] One way to show that you are receptive to mentally disabled students is to use welcoming language on your syllabus. Your institution might require you to put canned language on your syllabus about disability services. This language likely comes across as impersonal, like all of such statements I've seen. I suggest framing such statements with your own words, like this:

"[Your college] requires me to put this language on our syllabus, so I am including it here; you might find the information useful."

This sentence lets students know that the canned statement is not how *you* would write about disability—yet they still have access to the important data. Elsewhere on your syllabus—ideally on the first page— add a statement that is warm and welcoming about disability. Something like this:

If you are disabled, I welcome a conversation to discuss your learning needs. You do not need official disability status with our institution, and you do not need to disclose your disability to me. I want to make sure you succeed in our course.

Something that simple sends a big message. You welcome disabled students' presence, and you are willing to collaborate to build an accessible classroom.

Note that my suggested words don't mention "accommodations." The words specifically state that you are not going to require any official paperwork, nor are you only interested in "requirements." You are telling your students that the conversation will not be about the bare minimum required by law. No, it will be about what you can do to ensure your students get the best education you can give them. Accessible course design accounts for the presence of mentally disabled students, including the many students who are unable to get accommodations from campus disability services.

Accessible course design must account for the wide variety of mentally disabled students. Costa told me, "One of the first things we [faculty] need to do is to remember that the neurodiversity paradigm recognizes the wide variety of neurotypes in the human species." For example, students with autism, ADHD, anxiety, depression, and so forth might all have executive function challenges.[28] Despite these similarities, they all have different needs. Thus, Costa notes, "From a very practical standpoint, certain strategies work well for most, though not all, students." Because of the diversity even within each neurotype, using accessible course design becomes even more important for us as faculty.

Costa provides some general ideas for designing an accessible course, such as, "Put things in writing. Make instructions and expectations external and clear. Be concise and specific in your instructions." Importantly, Costa notes, consider yourself a collaborator in your mentally disabled students' education journey: "Always keep student agency at the forefront of your design decisions. Partner with students to get their needs met." This collaborative approach works with *all* students and can create a course with immense student buy-in.

Course design begins early, before the semester starts. I want to emphasize that I, too, have scrambled to put together a syllabus at the last minute. After all, I've taught as a contingent professor for twenty years, sometimes having courses dropped in my lap shortly before the semester begins—and recently, *after* the semester began. However, my own autistic brain demands organization—now, as a professor, and years ago, when I was a student. This organization includes clear course expectations, knowledge of what coursework is due when, and an understanding of how assignments affect student learning outcomes and grades. I can't teach amid chaos, and, in retrospect, I had trouble learning that way too.

Now I always present students with a well-written syllabus. My syllabus includes brief yet clear course expectations (including details about grading, attendance, and deadlines), well-designed assignments, and readings and assignments planned out on a schedule for the entire semester (with no TBDs in sight). My students always express their appreciation of my organization—*all* of my students. Creating a well-written syllabus also has made me a better teacher because such planning makes me conscious of what I'm teaching, why I'm teaching it, and how.

Imagine being a mentally disabled student who struggles with staying organized, with breaking big tasks into smaller tasks, or with sorting important information from less important information. Here are some suggestions for creating a syllabus that best communicates with mentally disabled students so that they can succeed:

- Make your syllabus an organized tool that gives them plenty of time to plan ahead and sort information by degrees of importance.
- Use good document design that makes information easy to locate. Use meaningful headings that are easy to find. Use one easy-to-read font. Use short paragraphs.

- Distinguish must-read information from information that students only need to reference. You can label one part of your syllabus as "Primary" and another as "Secondary."
- Plan your course schedule before the semester begins so that the second half is not filled with stressful TBDs. (An added benefit: you will think through your course and its purpose before stepping foot in the classroom—making your course stronger and easier to teach.)
- Keep your course management software thoughtfully structured, rather than using it as a disorganized file dump. Once you have a good structure, you can export it and use it from semester to semester. (This is what I do.)
- Make the tone of your syllabus explicitly welcoming and supportive of mentally disabled students and, as I suggest earlier, add language to make it so.

If you need to adjust your schedule later, that's okay. Just give your students plenty of notice and do it in an organized fashion. What is not okay is disorganization, vagueness about assignments or course expectations, and high-stakes, last-minute changes. Mentally disabled students suffer most under these conditions—but *all* of your students suffer some.

If you design and teach an accessible course, your mentally disabled students will feel welcome and will believe you want them to succeed. As Garcia writes, "The main reason autistic people fear asking for accommodations [is because] it feels as if we're seeking out special treatment and that we're the problem."[29] In reality, Garcia points out, "asking for help is about addressing structural problems." An accessible classroom is one antidote to these structural problems. As autistic professor Maggie Coughlin writes, "The things those of us on the spectrum need will benefit everyone, as well: more precise communication, well-organized material, clearly defined expectations and rules, fewer distractions, and acceptance. Just imagine how much more peaceful and effective your classes could be."[30] Seriously: imagine with me. And let's make it a reality.

13

Front-Line Faculty

A certain subset of faculty carry a heavier burden caring for our students' mental health, a burden that goes beyond what most consider "teaching." These "front-line faculty," as I call them, have close contact with students and are therefore in a position to notice—and do something about—students' mental health struggles.[1] They are the people whom students turn to first when they are struggling. For this reason, front-line faculty bear an immense emotional burden.

This is not a COVID phenomenon, although their workload has grown during the pandemic. As I wrote in 2017, "As educators, we are on the front lines of students' mental-health issues, and we are often called upon, in the heat of the moment, to listen to what may be shocking revelations from our students—about their mental health, addiction, trauma, or more."[2] I wrote those words as a contingent faculty member, as a woman, as a disabled teacher, and as a teacher of first-year, small-section, mandatory writing courses. All of these intersecting identities put me on the front line—my various vulnerabilities combined with my students' access to me.

Front-line labor in higher education is distributed unequally.[3] First, front-liners tend to occupy lower-tiered positions in institutional hierarchies, such as contingent faculty positions with little job security. Second, they tend to teach introductory or low-status courses with fewer students, so their students get to know them well. At the undergraduate level, front-liners teach first-year composition and small sections or lab sections that support large lectures (which are taught by tenured abdicators). In law schools, they teach first-year legal writing or in law clinics. And so on. Third, front-liners are professors from marginalized groups who are expected to bear the burden of advising students from their own marginalized groups—even if those students are not their own. This advising work is not remunerated, and it often eats into time when a professor would be planning courses or working on research. Most front-line professors are there because institutional circumstances require it. They cannot opt out. (Note that some of the professors who are pressured to be on the front line would have chosen to work there; the point is that they do not have an option.)

Who is not on the front line? These "tenured abdicators" tend to share three traits. First, they tend to be tenured professors with good job security. Second, they tend to teach large lecture classes, where it is difficult for students to form close bonds with them unless the professor chooses to let them. Third, they tend not to be members of marginalized groups. Because of their status in the institutional employment hierarchy and because of the courses they teach, these professors do not need to learn students' names or engage with them. They might meet students only during their brief office hours. Because professors tend to be white and male, marginalized students don't turn to them for mentoring, because these students prefer mentors who look like them or because they hope (and expect) a female professor will be more nurturing. Finally, tenured abdicators receive no institutional punishment for opting out of front-line labor. Indeed, they often opt out of other departmental work as well, such as committee work, a phenomenon called "social loafing."[4] Some faculty who need not do front-line work opt in to the front line. These faculty are rare, but they do exist.

Law professor Meera E. Deo, who studies both the stratification of labor in law schools and mental health, uses the term "vulnerable law teachers" to describe a group that lines up well with front-line faculty.[5] Vulnerable law teachers include "the overlapping categories of caregivers, untenured faculty, women of color, and white women."[6] If you are vulnerable, as characterized by Deo, chances are you are on the front line—because of your very vulnerability. Other front-line faculty include advisers, who frequently end up supporting students emotionally and academically.

Being on the front line is emotionally draining. Not only must front-line faculty carry out our regular responsibilities, but we must also do unrecognized and unremunerated care work for our students who desperately need it. To make matters worse, front-line faculty look around and see our colleagues, ones who have greater institutional power and make a whole lot more money, opting out of this work—shirking all responsibilities for their students' mental health. This shirking not only adds to the burden front-line faculty bear but also harms our students because many of their professors—whom they look to for mentorship—pull away from them.

I see two possible ways to lighten the load that front-line faculty bear. The first is to share the load equally so that all faculty on campus tend to our students' mental health. (I leave it up to administrators wiser than I am to figure out how to implement this solution.) To me, this is the ideal solution because it means that every professor would have the chance to get to know their students as whole people—or at all, given that many professors spend little time even talking to their students. Plus, the emotional load that each professor bears would become minimal because the load would be spread so widely.

The second way to lighten the load on front-line faculty would be to accept that front-line faculty are going to bear the emotional load—and then compensate them for it and give them the time to do it. Recognizing that they spend a large amount of time doing student carework means paying them to do this work (a salary increase) and creating time for it (via course release). Both are necessary to prevent burnout.

If you are on the front lines, I recommend mitigating the strain on yourself. You can do so while still caring for your students. The typical way front-line faculty encounter students who are struggling with their mental health is disruptive and draining. Usually, it goes like this: A student comes to your office—perhaps during office hours, or perhaps when you are working in your office at other times. The student is in obvious distress, so you stop your work. You listen empathetically to the student, taking on part of their burden. Then you help the student problem-solve, figuring out what services or extra classroom support they need, if any. Essentially, your time with the student involves triage, diagnosis, and treatment. This work is, in a word, exhausting.

But our students are not to blame for these problems. They know little about the structure of higher education, how some faculty bear greater burdens than others, about pay disparities and labor disparities, about how race and gender affect work and pay distribution. In addition to my advice here, I advocate sharing this information with our students.[7]

Mental Health Communities

One way to make your work easier as front-line faculty is to create "student mental health communities." In these communities, students learn to trust one another with their mental health struggles, relieving the burden on you. You are no longer the only person students come to for assistance—especially when that assistance is just a nonjudgmental ear. But you must cultivate these communities and the trust they're founded upon. Here are some suggestions for creating these communities to help your students learn to support each other so that you are not the only one they can turn to for help.

During the fall semester of 2021, tragedy struck our campus in the form of multiple student suicides and suicide attempts. During our first class meeting after another student death, the air was full of tension and grief. I knew that the ethical thing to do was to directly acknowledge our campus mental health tragedies. I would break my students' trust if I ignored their struggles. The best solution I could think of was to tackle the issue head on. For me, that meant sharing my own story, in particular about the depression I had dealt with most recently. I stood in the front of the room, facing my seminar students. I started by asking, with a smile, "Do you guys google your professors? Like, have you googled me?"

They shook their heads.

I was incredulous. "Man, if I were in school now, I would google all of my professors." I laughed, but I was also serious. Researching my professors' identities was much harder twenty years ago.

Also, I'd hoped that at least some of them would have researched me on the internet. What I was about to say would have been so much easier if they had already known about my mental disability. Instead, I had to start cold.

I said, "I want to talk to you about mental health after everything that has happened over the past few days."

One student was making eye contact with me while his fingers were moving on his laptop keyboard.

I nodded at him and smiled. "Are you googling me now?"

We both laughed. Of course he was.

"Good," I said to him. "Everything I'm about to tell you is out there." I waved my hand to encompass *out there*. On the internet, there was plenty of public information about my mental disabilities—in stories I'd written, in interviews I'd given, in tweets, Instagram posts, and more. In fact, outside the walls of our institution, I'd been very open about my mental disabilities.

Even so, I was nervous about what I was about to say.

I leaned back against the whiteboard. "I have bipolar disorder and I'm autistic. A while ago, I nearly died by suicide. And sometimes, I get severely depressed."

I was nervous my students would think less of me, that I had lost credibility as a professor. That all of the things I knew to be true about the stigma against mental disability in higher education would harm my relationship with my students. Margaret Price writes in her book *Mad at School*, "Persons with mental disabilities are presumed not to be competent, nor understandable, nor valuable, nor whole . . . The failure to make sense, as measured against and by those with 'normal' minds, means a loss of personhood."[8] I had never stood in front of my own students and told them I was mentally disabled. What if everything went wrong?

I continued, telling the story of how I almost hadn't been their professor that fall because I'd been so depressed over the summer. Then the professor who'd been scheduled to teach my class in my place backed out right before the semester. "So the law school reached out to me at the last minute," I told them. "I felt healthy again, and here I am." By telling them about my own recent depression, I wanted to show my students that stigma is a powerful thing, how it instills fear in the hearts of the stigmatized, even those who *know* that mental disability is nothing to be ashamed of—like me.

I said, "Your lives are impossible right now. I'm so sorry. There are people who want to help you, and I'm one of them. You can always come to me. I know what it's like to feel like everything is dark. I promise."

Then I stopped talking at them and asked if anyone had any questions. "Even really personal ones," I joked.

I waited for a while, giving my students plenty of space to think. Eventually, one student said, with deep sincerity, "Thank you." There were murmurs of agreement.

After class, two students hung around and thanked me in private for sharing my story. Then, a few days later, I received a direct message from a student, printed here with permission:

I just wanted to thank you again for being vulnerable with us last week. If those in positions of power, leadership, etc. over us aren't vulnerable to talk about hard things then why would we ever be?

The student's words evoked what I had tried to do in class: to show my own vulnerability to them so that they could see that being vulnerable need not be scary under the proper circumstances, and that it might even be helpful. I tried to create an environment that fought back against stigma, where students felt comfortable talking to each other even if they did not feel comfortable talking to me.

After that day, and for the rest of the semester, I collaborated with my students on ways that I could make the course logistically easier for them. We collaborated on a method to take the final exam that eased the logistical burden almost entirely. The course remained intellectually demanding, but my students did not have to fret about, for example, whether the intricacies of our institution's course management software were going to trip them up.

Not every contingent professor can disclose their mental disabilities the way I did. In fact, I have, over and over, advised against disclosing mental disabilities in the workplace, especially in higher education, unless you have bulletproof job security.[9] For all of the reasons Margaret Price describes, most should not. Higher education, as an institution, is not yet a place inclusive enough for faculty to disclose their mental disabilities. But even if you do not share your personal story (or if you do not have one to share), you can still talk about mental health with your students.

To facilitate a mental health community among your students, I recommend doing a "mental health acknowledgment" every class, for two or three minutes, nothing more. These acknowledgments will become easier to do with repetition, for you and for your students. You can start by acknowledging that their lives are hard. Just saying the words out loud can do a lot for your students by showing that you see them: "I want to acknowledge those of you who are struggling right now. If you are, it is real. It is hard, and I'm sorry." The first time you say these words, you might not feel ready to ask any questions. That's okay. It's enough that your students heard you.

The next class meeting, say the words again. After you finish speaking, be silent, giving your students time to think. Then ask: "What has been hard on campus these past few days?" With this question, you aren't asking your students to pour out their hearts about personal stuff. You're asking a general question about life on campus. After you pose the question, wait—longer than you think. Your students are likely un-accustomed to talking about mental health topics.

Finally, start the next class meeting with a simple acknowledgment, followed by a check-in. Say the words, "I'm doing . . ." and an honest description of your mental health situation, then ask, "How are you do-ing?" If there are campus events that deserve attention (like the one I addressed with my class), address them directly. Then give them space to speak. Don't worry—you are not running a group therapy session—just a place where students can talk about hard things. Give them plenty of opportunities to learn to talk about such taboo subjects.

Every time you talk with your students about mental health, you destigmatize it, give your students a way to talk about their own strug-gles, and build a stronger community. By creating an inclusive space—a classroom that celebrates mental disability and supports mental health struggles—you create a space in which you and your students can push back against the stigma against mental disabilities that stops people from seeking help for their mental health struggles.

In the end, having a class-wide discussion about the mental health struggles your students face will likely decrease the number of students who need to come talk to you in private. Not only are you giving stu-dents space to share their worries in class, but you will also have culti-vated a supportive community among them. You are showing them that they are not alone in how they are feeling. They have each other.

I am learning that one of the most important things I can do as a professor is acknowledge to my students when things are difficult, for them and for me. When things are hard, acknowledging the hardness, saying the words out loud, can make a big difference.

Group Office Hours

In addition to the classroom acknowledgments described above, you can hold group, rather than individual, office hours—online or in per-son. Law professor and academic support expert Sarah J. Schendel has pointed out that individual office hours (in particular, online office hours) can intimidate some students, and she suggests offering group office hours.[10] I suggest deliberately creating online group office hours, which will facilitate your mental health community, build bonds between your students, and reduce the number of hours you must meet with students, because you aren't meeting with them individually.

Alexa Z. Chew, a law professor at the University of North Carolina School of Law, used Zoom to hold chat sessions with current and former students during the COVID pandemic. Her goal was to support her students and help them build community. (Professor Chew is front-line faculty: she teaches a first-year writing course every semester, she is Asian American, she is a woman, and she is contingent faculty.) Professor Chew sent an email to all of her students, past and present, who were still students at her institution, stating that she would be holding chat sessions with students in groups ranging in size from two to eight. She then created a signup using her meeting software. The spots quickly filled.

Students across all years wanted to chat. In the larger online groups, some students chose not to speak but listened to others share their stories. In the smaller groups, students could have Professor Chew's close attention. In the end, Professor Chew's students were able to build community by meeting one another in a non-classroom environment. The chats enabled them to create valuable connections at a time when connections have been so hard to come by.

When you nurture community among your students, they have others to turn to besides you. If front-line faculty spend time cultivating student communities, we will create a new, more powerful front line that supports students' mental health struggles. This front line is less burdensome on its faculty members because it is made up of fellow students who trust one another, forming an interlocking web of support.

Institutions Must Protect Front-Line Faculty

Institutions must fix the inequities that allow front-line work to be unevenly distributed, unacknowledged, and unremunerated. If deans and chairs cannot require all faculty to help students, they can require tenured abdicators to make their status transparent so that students know those professors are not available to help them with all aspects of their education. Right now, this unbalanced distribution of labor is invisible to our students, and to many professors. Making it visible will help front-line faculty understand whom they can lean on for assistance and help students know whom they can, and cannot, turn to for help.

For example, if a professor chooses to opt out of front-line work during office hours, institutions can choose to require them to make this information known to their students. Thus, tenured abdicators should be required to add a line to their syllabus like this:

> During my office hours, I am only available to discuss History of the Civil War [or whatever course the professor teaches]. I am not available to discuss any topic concerning your mental health or well-being.

It is important to inform students that they cannot turn to tenured abdicators for help in order to protect their mental health. What if a student were to turn to a professor for help and be painfully rebuffed? After such a rejection, the student may not seek help from faculty again, fearing another rejection—which could have tragic results.

Granted, such a syllabus requirement is unlikely to happen—despite my earnestness in suggesting it—because administrators are unlikely to require it. But here's a tactic that journalism professor Teresa Heinz Housel suggested to me: we can advise our students to compile information about faculty who are more accessible and those who are more closed off.[11] Front-line faculty can make this suggestion to our students when we help them form their mental health communities, saying something like this: "Some professors aren't open to discussing your mental health and well-being. As you discover who these professors are, crowdsource this information among yourselves." Empower students to discover which professors are unhelpful, even hostile, to their mental health struggles.

Our students are not only in college to grow intellectually, but to grow as whole persons. Thus, part of our role as faculty is to cultivate the whole person. Perhaps, at an administrative level, it is more practical for only certain faculty to be doing such work. In that case, those faculty should be compensated for that work. Administrators can provide support to front-line faculty via methods such as decreased committee work (and other service work) and course releases. If an institution is struggling to find the budget to justify supporting front-line faculty, consider this: surely doing so is less expensive than losing hundreds of students (and their money) to attrition because their mental health struggles were ignored.

Front-line faculty cannot save institutions. They must save themselves. The good news is that institutions do have the power to help front-line faculty. Recognizing the labor front-line faculty do and providing them with relief will go a long way to retaining faculty, increasing morale, preventing burnout, and ensuring our students receive the support they need.

14

Procrastination and Compassion

One recent semester, I had a student who just could not seem to get his writing assignments turned in on time. I knew that he wasn't a bad student: he was participating in class, giving feedback to his classmates during writing workshops, and generally doing the things that hard-working students do.

But his assignments were late, and some of them were missing entirely. So, after class one day, I privately asked him about the missing work. First, I said, "You do not have to share your personal life with me. I respect your privacy." I firmly believe that no student should have to hand over their secrets in order to receive academic support from faculty. At the same time, I wanted him to know that I would provide a sympathetic ear. Therefore, I said, "But I'm happy to listen."

He chose to share with me some personal struggles. After he shared them, he told me, urgently, "I'm not making excuses."

"I know that," I said. He wasn't. Giving reasons is not making excuses. Reasons are unavoidable events that cause effects. Reasons include a difficult pregnancy, the birth of a child, or the death of a loved one. Reasons are illness, physical or mental.

The struggles he shared were serious, and I never would have known about them if he hadn't told me, given his cheerful in-class demeanor. I could not have imagined all of the things he kept hidden beneath that veneer. The hiding alone must have been exhausting.

We discussed his late assignments, and then I said, "You tell me. What is a deadline that you can meet?"

He looked at me with surprise, as though he had never had a professor ask him that question before. Perhaps he hadn't. Then we collaborated

on a deadline that worked for him (instead of me handing him an arbitrary deadline that didn't account for the struggles he was facing). Re-
markably, the one he chose was way shorter than the one I would have
given him.

After we finished, he had an empowered look on his face that told
me I had helped him learn a valuable lesson about managing time,
planning ahead, and standing up for himself when he is overwhelmed.
Indeed, as law professor and academic support expert Sarah J. Schendel
notes, teaching students how to ask for extensions is just as important
as having deadlines.[1] The two—extensions and deadlines—are insepa-
rable in the real world, so they both must be taught in school. Students
who are overwhelmed, like my student was, will procrastinate; it is inevitable. If we don't learn how procrastination works and what to do about
it, we will face broken deadlines, shoddy work, and anxious students.

What Is Procrastination?

For psychologists, procrastination is "the voluntary delay of an intended
act despite the awareness that this needless delay will be detrimental in
the longer term."[2] Procrastination is thus something that the procrastinator is aware that they are doing, and that they are also aware will hurt
them. Students who procrastinate are not lazy, or bad students, or poor
planners. They are struggling with a real psychological problem. I admit
that until I began this research, I did not understand the extent of the
problem. I believed that procrastination was laziness. I know now, as an
absolute fact, that procrastination is not about willpower.

Procrastination's Causes and Effects

Many of our students struggle with procrastination. Some always have,
and many professors have blamed them for being lazy or poor planners.
Some students are struggling with procrastination for the first time,
brought on by the new stress of college life.

Psychologist Devon Price, an expert on procrastination, has famously
proclaimed that "laziness does not exist."[3] According to Price, procrastination is driven either by "anxiety about . . . not being 'good enough'"
or by confusion about what the first steps of the task are. Contrary to
popular belief, Price points out, "procrastination is more likely when the

task is meaningful and the individual cares about doing it well." When a person cares deeply about a task, the person can become paralyzed by the fear of failure.

A recent study on procrastination found a link between feeling awful about yourself and procrastination. Procrastinators "have a chronic tendency to cognitively dwell on their dysphoric feelings [feelings of profound unhappiness] and on negative self-relevant information."[4] In other words, procrastinators chronically focus on their bad feelings about their lives in general and on bad feelings about themselves. Together, these bad feelings create chronic self-doubt, which leads to procrastination.

In times of crisis, say, during a worldwide pandemic, one might have stronger feelings of dysphoria—profound unhappiness—than normal. The same holds true in times of personal crisis. Negative thoughts about our personal experiences spill over into negative thoughts about ourselves and our ability to get things done. After all, in difficult times, it is easy to feel helpless. And when all of these bad feelings converge, it is easy to procrastinate.

Indeed, the study noted that procrastinators also have really bad feelings about their "self-efficacy."[5] Self-efficacy is the belief in your ability to get something done. If you have strong self-efficacy, when faced with a challenging task, you feel confident in your ability to accomplish whatever the task throws your way. If you have low self-efficacy, you will doubt your ability to accomplish the task.

Thus, if a student who ordinarily has strong self-efficacy has a paper due tomorrow, and they have spent two weeks unable to get a single word down on the page, they will start to doubt their ability to succeed in any college course at all. That is, they transfer their negative belief about the paper to other, completely unrelated activities in their life, like their ability to get the laundry done. Then the laundry piles up, creating a self-fulfilling prophecy. Procrastination tanks self-efficacy, and poor self-efficacy fuels procrastination.

Thus, you can think of procrastination as a cycle. Because of our stressful environment, or our own psychiatry, or our awful life events, or all of the above, we feel poorly. Because we feel poorly, we cannot do our work, and that makes us feel worse. Perhaps we even develop depression or anxiety. Because we are depressed or anxious, we certainly cannot work.

It is unsurprising then that procrastination researchers have found that "procrastination and depression were linked significantly."[6] Indeed, these researchers found "the association between depression and procrastination-related thoughts was stronger" than they had expected it to be. Thus, if a student of yours is struggling with procrastination, there is a chance that they are also struggling with depression. (The same goes for you too.)

Procrastination and Anxiety

Procrastination and anxiety are also linked. To paraphrase what Devon Price mentioned, if a student feels anxious about a task, they are more likely to procrastinate. Take in this scenario: Imagine you were a successful student in high school. You developed good study habits and routines, and you followed them. But coming to college upended your routines, as it does for many students when they leave behind their support systems and enter an environment with new and complicated rules. You start to worry; you start to worry more as your academic success starts to drop because you spend so much time fretting. You try to keep your grades up, but it costs you a lot of lost sleep and long hours to do so.

You can't relax. You try to build new routines, but you can't do that either. You don't know why. When you go to the library to write a paper and someone is sitting in your favorite spot, you get upset and leave, unable to concentrate on your paper at all. You try to sleep, but you are too wound up about your inability to work. Because you didn't sleep, you are too fatigued the next day to finish the paper, so you get a cup of coffee. But the coffee doesn't help; in fact, it just makes you more anxious and irritable. You can't concentrate, and your mind keeps wandering. You get frustrated and give up, turning in work you are ashamed of. The next time you try to work, all you can think about is that terrible work you turned in last time, and you are worried you will do the same thing again. You are worried that you are a terrible student, that your whole life you were just faking it. You spiral, down, down, and down.

This student is getting devoured by anxiety disorders and, like so many of their peers, they are blaming themself for its symptoms. They have not, and likely will not, reach out for mental health care because they simply do not have the knowledge about anxiety to understand what is happening to them. Institutional factors created the fertile ground in which student anxiety disorders grow. Institutional solutions are required to help heal it. For example, institutions can disseminate knowledge across campus about what anxiety disorders look like and how students can seek help; they can educate faculty about how to help students with anxiety disorders—with compassion rather than punishments. Instead, what frequently happens is the student guts it out alone, and then faces harsh punishment for procrastination, one of the few visible outcomes of their anxiety disorder. As you can imagine, such punishments only make things worse.

Self-Compassion

Luckily, there are solutions that can break the cycle of procrastination, anxiety/depression, and low self-efficacy. Procrastinators, the study notes, "tend to be low in self-compassion."[7] However, "individuals who reported high procrastination but who also forgave themselves (an act of self-compassion) were less likely to procrastinate on the same task in the future than those who reported a lack of forgiveness."[8] The answer, then, is to cultivate self-compassion among our students.

What is self-compassion? According to the study, self-compassion is "an emotionally positive view whereby individuals feel warmth and understanding towards themselves when faced with life difficulties."[9] When you practice self-compassion, when challenges arise or when you feel like you are going to fail (or already have), you deliberately cut yourself a break and forgive yourself. Kristin D. Neff, psychology researcher and expert in self-compassion, explains in her groundbreaking 2003 article that self-compassion works by first welcoming one's struggles instead of avoiding them: "Self-compassion . . . involves being touched by and open to one's own suffering, not avoiding or disconnecting from it."[10] Thus, self-compassion requires acknowledging your mistakes or other bad things happening in your life and allowing yourself to feel "kindness and caring" for yourself—the way you would treat a good friend who was struggling with similar things. If you treat yourself with this sort of kindness, you will "generat[e] the desire to alleviate one's suffering and to heal oneself with kindness." Instead of running yourself down with negative thoughts and making the bad thing worse, you will feel more positive about your ability to make things better and to fix whatever problem you are facing.

Self-compassion, according to Neff, helps us avoid being judgmental about our mistakes. It does so by framing "one's experience . . . as part of the larger human experience."[11] When we can see that we are not alone in making mistakes and failing, it is easier to forgive ourselves for making those mistakes and for those failures. Self-compassion puts our own mistakes into perspective, so to speak, not to minimize the pain we are feeling—failure *hurts*—but to help us see that we are not the only people on planet Earth who have ever failed. If we can help our students understand these truths, we can help them stop procrastinating. In fact, Neff's research has shown the connection between self-compassion and academic motivation in college students.[12] In a 2005 study, she and her team found a connection between self-compassion and the ability of students to cope with failure. For students, her research showed, self-compassion created intrinsic motivation and helped alleviate anxiety.[13]

Practicing Self-Compassion

How do we teach our students to have self-compassion and overcome procrastination? In their research, Neff and her team note that professors play an important role in helping students who are struggling, by encouraging self-compassion "in conjunction with an emphasis on mastery rather than performance goals."[14] How, exactly, can we teach our students self-compassion when they are struggling with procrastination? Neff describes three facets of self-compassion:

(1) "Self-kindness," which is "extending kindness and understanding to oneself rather than harsh judgment and self-criticism."
(2) "Common humanity," which is "seeing one's experiences as part of the larger human experience rather than seeing them as separating and isolating."
(3) "Mindfulness," which is "holding one's painful thoughts and feelings in balanced awareness rather than over-identifying with them." [15]

These are large-scale concepts. As faculty, however, we can use this framework to guide our particular student interactions.

Self-kindness: If we hear students running themselves down with harsh self-judgment, we can help them understand that procrastination is wrongly seen, as Schendel puts it, "as a personality trait or individual failure, rather than as a broader issue of misunderstanding or underestimating what the task will entail."[16] Pointing out this misunderstanding of the nature of procrastination can help a student understand that procrastination is not a character flaw that they can never fix. Instead, we, and our students, should understand that procrastination is frequently linked to "planning fallacy," as Schendel explains, which is the "strong bias to underestimate how long it will take to complete almost any task."[17] Planning fallacy is not only common but it can be overcome. Point them to resources for how to do so—and if we need those resources ourselves, we can ask our institution's teaching and learning resources center for help.

Common humanity: If a student suggests that they are the only one who is a failure, we can point out that this is not the case. Explain that many students struggle with planning, and that the student is not alone. Emphasize that failure is a common human experience and not something to be ashamed of. As law professor and student support specialist Kaci Bishop explains, there is a strong connection between perfectionism, fear of failure, and procrastination.[18] She points out how "those with perfectionist tendencies are more likely to see even small mistakes or setbacks as significant failures."[19] Worse, she notes that "in the face of repeated failure (or perceived failure)," some students "may spiral into feeling guilt and shame, as well as anxiety, depression, and anger."[20] These feelings of guilt and shame are not unique to an individual, but shared by everyone who strives to do well.

Mindfulness: If a student overly focuses on their failures, while at the same time blowing off their successes, we can help them learn how to celebrate their successes, ensuring a balanced perspective. Celebrate student wins, no matter how small, during class time or when evaluating student work. It is unlikely that our students are celebrating them enough.

As faculty, we must also have compassion for ourselves for failing to meet deadlines, for feeling too exhausted to work some days, and for not having the energy to do every small thing that needs doing. We can model this good behavior for our students by doing it ourselves.

15

Teaching Accessibly/Inclusively

In Part II of this book, I have been building toward one simple call: we must teach accessibly and inclusively to ensure that all of our students have the opportunity to learn. As I have shown throughout this book, inclusion of mental disability on campus counters the stigma that mentally disabled students and faculty face. Breaking down that stigma helps all students and faculty who are struggling with their mental health, because it makes it easier for them to ask for help. In the classroom, accessible/inclusive teaching reduces barriers to learning for all students, not just those with disabilities recognized by the disability services office.

Although the call is simple, teaching accessibly/inclusively can seem intimidating to those who are unfamiliar with how to do so. Teaching accessibly/inclusively improves learning outcomes for all students and across all courses, and it will also make every professor a better teacher. This is a big claim; nevertheless, it is true. In this final chapter, I provide actionable steps to help faculty implement accessible/inclusive teaching strategies.

I refer to my teaching style as "accessible/inclusive"—both terms, together. When professors think of students with disabilities, they think of accommodations. But accessibility is not the same as the accommodation of disability. Accommodations are special exceptions made for one disabled person, and they require the disabled person to jump through lots of administrative—and costly—hoops to get them. Accessibility is the existence of a space that is hospitable to and usable by all disabled people. There are no gatekeepers to an accessible space. Thus, accessible teaching presumes that disabled students are always present and teaches with them in mind.

Inclusion of mentally disabled people means removing any burdens to allow them to join a community that has previously stigmatized them. Inclusion does not put the onus on mentally disabled people to join in; instead inclusion means taking active steps to welcome them. Mentally disabled students are already present, in great numbers, in our classrooms. The onus is on the institution, and on faculty, to include them with our teaching practices.

Guiding Principles

I provide three guiding principles to teaching accessibly/inclusively: (1) agency, (2) empathy, and (3) accessibility for everyone.

Agency. Agency means students have the power of self-determination. Agency is often diametrically opposed to many toxic teaching tactics used by professors today—including those who do not even realize that they are using them. These toxic tactics create hurdles that infantilize students and reveal professors' deep mistrust of them.[1] Disability studies scholar Jay Dolmage notes that, in a classroom accessibility context, agency allows students "to have a shaping role in the event or class, as well as the right to define [their] own identity and involvement."[2] When professors collaborate with students on classroom accommodations, for example, we give our students agency.

Empathy. When I talk about teaching with empathy, I am talking, in part, about what Professor Catherine J. Denial calls "kindness." How does kindness look in practice? According to Denial, it is "two simple things: believing people, and believing in people."[3] Every teaching practice I suggest requires that you have faith in your students, that you believe that they are honest, and that you believe that they are deserving of agency.

Accessibility for Everyone. To state that accessibility is "for everyone" is not about diminishing the importance of accessibility for disabled people; it is the opposite. It is the recognition that disabled people are everywhere, always. Therefore, we must make accessibility a practice by everyone, for everyone and counteract ableist teaching practices whenever possible.

With these three guiding principles in mind—agency (as opposed to toxic rigor), kindness (as opposed to lack of faith), and accessibility for everyone (as opposed to ableism)—let's look at how to teach accessibly/inclusively.

Recognize, and Stop, Toxic Rigor

Rigor angsters fear that our academic standards are on a downward spiral, and their solution is toxic rigor. Rigor angst has come to the fore during the pandemic, but you do not have to look very hard to see that it has always been a higher education bogeyman. In fact, Denial's "Pedagogy of Kindness," a response to rigor angst, was written in 2019. Whenever toxic rigor comes to the forefront of pedagogy debates, we can embrace the opportunity to quash it once and for all.

Toxic rigor increases "logistical rigor" in a course, to paraphrase history professor Kevin Gannon, which is coursework that does little to increase a student's learning and a lot to get in the way of it.[4] Logistical rigor creates what I call "bad-hard" coursework. Compare logistical rigor with "intellectual rigor," which challenges students to explore complex ideas and refine their own thinking. Intellectual rigor is "good-hard" coursework.

Examples of bad-hard coursework include mandatory attendance with punitive consequences, banning laptops and other assistive technology, refusing to grant reasonable extensions, and any other logistical hurdles that are detached from the actual learning of the course material. Bad-hard coursework takes away student agency and infantilizes students; it is the opposite of empathetic pedagogy because it is built on mistrust. Furthermore, it is an ableist way to teach.

Rigor angster Jonathan Malesic, in his 2022 opinion piece in the *New York Times* ("My College Students Are Not OK"), claims the easing of bad-hard coursework caused a breakdown in student learning during the pandemic.[5] After recounting how student performance had fallen off sharply since the return to campus after the pandemic shutdown, he noted that, with regards to "attendance, late assignments, quality of in-class discussion . . . [his students] performed worse than any students I had encountered in two decades of teaching." One professor told Malesic that, on their first exam of fall 2020, they saw "the worst performance I'd ever seen on a test." Another professor told him that "the students in her classroom often met her questions with blank stares." What caused this loss of good student performance? According to Malesic, the culprits were distance learning and soft course expectations. (Did he miss the part where there was a worldwide pandemic?) Malesic's solution? Rigorous course expectations (that is, more bad-hard coursework) and mandatory in-person learning (which is a type of bad-hard coursework).

When faced with students who are doing the "worst" ever in school, during a worldwide crisis unprecedented in their lifetimes, I wonder: How does a professor fail to be concerned that their students' poor performance might be caused by the compounding trauma of the ongoing crisis? How does a professor conclude that treating students "harder" is the right approach to help these traumatized students?

The answer is: I have no idea. I do know that if I were met by blank stares in a classroom, I would not blame too much Zoom (as Malesic does). Instead, I would worry in equal parts about my own pedagogy and my students' mental health. But not Malesic or his colleagues. Malesic acknowledges that "the pandemic certainly made college more challenging for students." However, he gives these challenges only passing attention. Instead, he blames the easing of bad-hard coursework for poor student performance: "Over the past two years, compassionate faculty members . . . have introduced recorded lectures, flexible attendance and deadline policies, and lenient grading." Decreasing bad-hard work, according to Malesic, caused a "learning breakdown." Bizarrely, Malesic manages to make "compassionate" sound like a dirty word. (Compare Malesic's language to rigor angster Deborah J. Cohan's negative portrayal of the "grace and compassion police" in Chapter 11, "Rigor Angst.")[6] A "pedagogy of kindness," to use Denial's term, could not be further from the pedagogy of professors who believe kindness is going to be the downfall of the US education system.

Malesic's rigor angst is not an outlier; it is representative of its type. Rigor angster professors, it seems, want someone to blame for their students' academic struggles, so they blame their students for not trying hard enough. They blame other professors for being too kind. Rigor angsters assume their students are trying to cheat by asking for extensions; they assume their students are lying when they say they need to miss class. In this vein, Malesic wraps up his piece with the words of a colleague who told him that "we do [students] a disservice when we presume they're too mentally ill or too traumatized to function." Setting aside how counterfactual this argument is (many of our students are, indeed, mentally ill and traumatized), another underlying problem with this essay and those like it is how patronizing it is. Rather than treating students as agents of their own education and worthy of our trust, Malesic treats them as children in need of discipline.

As the pandemic has brought to light, Malesic's way of thinking is pervasive. As with anything that is culturally entrenched and rendered invisible by its pervasiveness, Malesic's thoughts on attendance, deadlines, and more are likely ones you or your colleagues agree with, if only slightly. It is time for us to rethink everything about how we teach. It is time to root out toxic rigor everywhere.

Avoid Laptop Bans

Laptop bans are infantilizing, show a lack of faith in students, and are ableist—they fail completely when it comes to teaching accessibly/inclusively.

The debate over laptop bans seems to rise from the dead every August before the start of school. (Sometimes more frequently than that.) Professors who are all for banning laptops put forward the same tired arguments. Here they are, recounted neatly by attorney and disabled activist Matthew Cortland: students are distracted by the technology; students "hid[e] behind their laptop screens instead of engaging"; students will not learn to take notes properly, but will instead become "mere transcriptionists" when typing them; students are "not learning as well as those who take longhand notes."[6] Given all of these apparent problems, why not just ban laptops? Seems reasonable.

It is not. Banning laptops takes away student agency because students are no longer able to decide the best way to engage with course material—literally, they do not have the choice to decide how to take in what they are learning in class. Instead of being able to decide whether to type, students are forced to handwrite their notes.

Forcing students to handwrite does not guarantee better learning. There are a few handwriting-versus-laptops studies that anti-laptop professors rely upon to make their arguments, but these have been well debunked. The main study they point to, published in 2014 ("The Pen is Mightier Than the Keyboard"), suggests that students who took lecture notes longhand did better on a quiz given after a brief break.[7] But then, in 2021, new researchers replicated the study ("Don't Ditch the Laptops Just Yet").[8] In this study, the difference in performance between the laptop notetakers and the handwriting notetakers was not significant enough to "support the idea that longhand notetaking improves immediate learning."[9] In short, science does *not* support the notion that handwriting notes is (universally) better than typing them. Instead of telling our students what to do, we must empower our students to decide what is best for them.

Taking away laptops does not guarantee that students will stay engaged. In an article on laptop bans and ableism ("When You Talk About Banning Laptops, You Throw Disabled Students Under the Bus") Professor Jordynn Jack and I point out how the supposed lack of student engagement caused by laptops is a professor's problem to fix by teaching better: "The professor's job is not to lecture, but to guide and to gauge student understanding. Students no longer passively take notes as the professor drones on. They use laptops to actively engage with each other and the course content."[10] If a professor does not engage students, students will zone out whether they have laptops or not. If a professor lectures to a passive audience, students will be passive notetakers by necessity, whether they handwrite those notes or type them. Like many readers of this book, I did not have a laptop in college. In boring lectures, I zoned out, entertaining myself with a crossword puzzle or doodling. When taking notes in such classes, I frequently "merely" transcribed. The medium does not matter if the teaching is poor.

Laptop bans do one thing well: they show that professors lack trust in their students, specifically, trust that their students know how to use technology in the way that is best for them. In short, bans show a lack of faith in students. Instead of banning laptops, why not talk to students about effective notetaking, distractions, and technology? Many people, including me, are tempted away from the work they are supposed to be doing by the tantalizing presence of social media and messaging with friends. (I am tempted, right now, as I write these words.) Treat your students like the adults they are and talk frankly about how to avoid technological temptation and focus instead. Then, show your faith in them by letting them try on their own.

Finally, laptop bans are ableist. Denial writes: "Because I don't believe students with disabilities should have to out themselves, I no longer ban laptops in my classroom."[11] If there is a student using a laptop in a course with a laptop ban, every other student in that course knows they are disabled with a laptop accommodation. Cortland points out that when a professor tries to get around the ableism of laptop bans by having exceptions for disabled students, the professor "exposes disabled and neurodiverse students to resentment and harassment."[12] That is, other students treat the person who has the laptop accommodation poorly because they resent them for having a privilege that they do not. Cortland explains, regarding being outed by laptop bans, "Being singled out as different on the basis of a disability is often terrifying, isolating, and miserable."[13] Sure, other students should not be resentful of a disabled student who needs an accommodation. But their resentment is understandable inside an ableist classroom structure that makes having an accommodation (i.e., a laptop) a highly desirable privilege.

Rather than banning laptops, Jack and I suggest setting up a classroom that "create[s] an accessible environment for disabled students," one where "students can engage with the course, express themselves, and access course information in different ways: electronically, during in-class discussions, in writing, and more."[14] Why? This style of teaching creates accessibility for everyone—elevating pedagogy and elevating learning.

Set Deadlines and Teach How to Ask for Extensions

If we set deadlines in our courses, we must allow for extensions. Deadlines and extensions go hand-in-hand—especially in the so-called real world. (When was the last time *you* asked for an extension?) Most students believe that extensions are not ever an option, especially if they have been conditioned by our norms of toxic rigor, under which deadlines are never, ever to be broken. As history professor Ellen Boucher wrote back in 2016 ("It's Time to Ditch Our Deadlines"), "It's time we give our students the same respect and flexibility that we demand in our own careers."[15] To do so, we must teach the skill of asking for extensions.

You should consider the teaching of extensions as the teaching of an important skill, rather than, as Sarah J. Schendel puts it, "anticipating failure, dismissing the importance of deadlines, or creating a way to avoid planning ahead."[16] Schendel, a law professor and academic support expert, notes that teaching extensions "pushes students to think beyond the due date itself to explicitly examine what it will take to meet the deadline." Thus, teaching extensions teaches students how to plan ahead, not to avoid doing so.

But you might presume that your students already know how to ask for extensions. Many professors do. Recently, I was chatting with a fellow professor who teaches at a midsized private university in the South. Debating with me the merits of teaching extensions, she said, "But some of my students do a very good job asking for them."

I replied, "That's because they know how and because they were brave enough to try." I emphasized that knowing how is not innate but learned, explaining that some students may never have needed to ask for an extension before and some students have only been punished for asking for extensions, so they stopped.

My colleague had never considered that students would not know how to ask for extensions, and she is a smart, empathetic professor.

There are other benefits to teaching extensions. One of them is that it helps students avoid procrastination, as Schendel observes.[17] She points out the misconception that many professors have about procrastination: that students are lazy or disengaged. As research shows, "While many professors see procrastination as a lack of engagement with the material, it can also be a result of anxiety or fear of not meeting high standards."[18] If you believe in your students, you believe that they might very well be late with their work because they care too much, not because they do not care enough.

But many empathetic professors have given me feedback that flexible deadlines increase their own workload to such a degree that they struggle to keep up with the work. I talked about this topic with Professor Teresa Heinz Housel, an expert in mental health and higher education, who has a flexible deadline policy that also takes her own workload into account.[19] She explained her policy to me: "My students can choose to use an optional extension that does not hurt their grades. If they choose to use it, however, they receive no individual feedback." But students still receive feedback on their work. Housel told me, "I give the class collective feedback so these students do receive feedback on the assignment." Housel's policy protects the professor's time while giving students the flexibility to plan their workload. Housel has used it in both introductory and high-level courses with success. Policies such as these allow students to prioritize without punishing their good decisions with bad grades.

If you have mentally disabled students in your class, know that many of them benefit from both deadlines (which provide organization and structure) and extensions (which provide a buffer for any unforeseen challenges that a mentally disabled student might encounter). Autistic professor Lydia X. Z. Brown, in conversation with autistic author and advocate Eric Garcia, explains how she handles deadlines to account for her mentally disabled students: "I set very clear and specific deadlines for each of the [assignments] so that students who are very structure-oriented and deadline-oriented would have a clear set of feasible deadlines."[20] But at the same time, in Brown's courses, "there is no such thing as late work."[21] That means, for Brown, if a student can't finish an assignment by the deadline, "all that you have to do is tell me when you think you will get it done by and that's your new deadline." Many mentally disabled students who come to college and struggle, Brown explains, are told they're "not really struggling"; instead, they're "just being lazy" or "making excuses." You might believe the same thing and be hesitant to grant deadlines. Or you might feel the need to take off points for late work. Resist the urge to punish, and collaborate with your students instead.

Believe Students Who Need Absences

Difficult and unpredictable things happen to students and faculty alike. And when those things happen, sometimes students will need to be absent from class. Denial explains how she had to learn "to ease up, to let go of rigid control I'd tried to impose upon the classroom, and to make room for the unpredictable and unexpected."[22] Denial describes how her former attendance policy "made no room for the idea that my students were adults with complicated lives who would need to miss a class now and again." A punitive attendance policy creates bad-hard work— in particular, "attend class at all costs"—and sometimes those costs are high. This type of policy is driven by faculty fear that students are slack-offs who don't care about school. If we get to know our students, what we find is that students who miss class are typically doing so because they are overwhelmed, sick, or otherwise struggling.

A professor colleague of mine, Ariane (a pseudonym), recently recounted to me a story about a particularly cruel undergraduate professor.[23] At the time, Ariane's father was having an organ removed because of cancer. Ariane told her professor that she would need to miss a class meeting because of her father's surgery. During this class meeting, Ariane was supposed to give a presentation. Instead of excusing the absence and granting an extension on the presentation, the professor told Ariane that she would fail the assignment. Ariane replied with grim acceptance, "That's fine." Suddenly, after Ariane stated that she would accept the failing grade, the professor changed her tune, granting the excused absence. Ariane explained to me how the threat of the failing grade was a test, like Solomon threatening to split the baby. Ariane's acceptance of the punishment proved to her professor that she wasn't lying about her father's critical surgery. What a terrible trick for her professor to play.

Ariane also told me that prior to this request, she had never missed a class meeting. Despite her perfect attendance, the professor was still suspicious of her motives to be absent. Furthermore, even after hearing that her student was struggling with a seriously ill parent, the professor never asked if Ariane was doing okay. Ariane's well-being did not even ping the professor's radar.

Denial's pedagogy of kindness is instructive when it comes to absences: "When a student comes to me to say that their grandparent died, I believe them. When they email me to say they have the flu, I believe them. When they tell me they didn't have time to read, I believe them. When they tell me their printer failed, I believe them."[24] Does this unwavering belief in her students make Professor Denial a sucker? Not really. She knows "there's an obvious chance that I could be taken advantage of in this scenario, that someone could straight-up lie and get away with it." For Denial, the risk of the rare devious student (and they are rare) is worth the benefit to the rest of her students: "I have learned that I would rather take that risk [of being lied to] than make life more difficult for my students struggling with grief and illness, or even an over-packed schedule or faulty electronics." In the simplest terms, she presumes her students are innocent. She does not treat them all with suspicion because a few might be dishonest. Instead, she believes them—how radical. Professor of literature at Penn State University Michael Bérubé has a similar philosophy. In a recent essay ("Cut Students Some Slack Already"), he writes, regarding his liberal approach to absences:

Might there be some students who are taking advantage of this flexibility, students who just don't feel like getting out of their pajamas, students who don't want to walk across an icy, windswept campus, students who just stayed up too late last night doing whatever?

I have no doubt that there are. And I am not terribly bothered by this.[25]

I do think we should take attendance and help our students make it to class—for one important reason. Absences are a tool we can use to monitor our students' mental health. If a student misses class frequently, we should presume they are struggling in some fashion. Using the data the absences provide, we can reach out to a student, ask to speak with them about their absences, and check to make sure they're okay. A frequently absent student is likely not okay at all.

Here are some ideas for how to approach a student. First, do not force them to disclose their private issues, but do tell them that you are willing to listen if they would like to share. Second, tell them they can come to you if they need help finding helpful resources, such as a referral to campus counseling. Finally, tell them that you would like to collaborate on a plan for them to attend class, then do so.

If you presume a student means well, they will sense it and will want to do the right thing. It is a rare student who is just a jerk; I have had only a few in my decades of teaching. The vast majority who acted like jerks did so because they expected to be treated badly for their mistakes. Once I earned their trust, they opened up to me with enormous hearts. Treat a student kindly and help redirect them before they fall too far behind academically or mentally.

Another thing to consider: many of us have more power than we realize to determine who is officially "absent." For example, at my institution, attendance is "mandatory" unless an absence is deemed "excused." Despite being a contingent faculty member, I still have enormous control over what counts as an excused absence or even an absence at all. I can determine what extra work students need to do, if any, to transform an unexcused absence into an excused absence. These days, my students don't have to do much at all to be "present"—just turn in any assignments due, watch the class recording, and message me that they've done so.

But for some professors, managing attendance exceptions in this fashion can create extra labor—especially for contingent professors. I am deeply sympathetic about any extra work piled on contingent faculty, front-line faculty, and any faculty who are already overburdened managing student welfare. I understand that this kind of accessible/inclusive teaching work can seem really hard when institutions do not support you. One of the ways I got around the overwork problem was by letting go of control in the classroom. When I let go of the feeling of needing to monitor my students so closely, my workload lightened along with my anxiety. In short, if you can, stop penalizing absences altogether, and you will have a lot less work to do.

When you teach accessibly/inclusively, attendance is a tool: if a student is persistently absent, they are giving you a sign to intervene and help them—while still respecting their privacy. If a student needs to miss class occasionally, however, it is none of our business.

Share Class Recordings and Other Materials with All Students

Usually we reserve the sharing of class lecture recordings for the few to whom we are legally required to give them because of their accommodations. Instead, we should make our class recordings available to all of our students. Providing the recordings to all is teaching accessibly, benefiting all mentally disabled students, not just those who could afford to get official accommodations. If we use slide decks to teach, we should provide those as well. Our goal is to help our students succeed, not hoard our knowledge.

Some faculty have concerns about sharing their lecture recordings because it is an invasion of privacy or abuse of intellectual property, and I understand those concerns. In response to the privacy argument, I respond that the notetakers must also put down their pens if private information is being shared during a class discussion.

However, there are other valid privacy reasons to not share class recordings, ones that would apply even to mentally disabled students. For example, a student in the class, or the professor, might be in danger if their location were made public. (This happens more than you might imagine. It is why some of our students elect to have their information kept out of the university directory and to have their photographs removed from any campus websites.)

There are other problems with sharing class recordings. For instance, some schools do not allow professors to record their class meetings. Researchers have also expressed valid concerns that some professors and institutions use the sharing of class recordings as a stand-in for teaching accessibly.[26] That is, some professors think, "I've shared my lecture recordings. Therefore I'm teaching accessibly." But sharing lecture recordings is only a small piece of the accessibility puzzle.

Jordynn Jack, my colleague at UNC–Chapel Hill, shared with me an alternative to sharing class recordings to create an accessible/inclusive course.[27] She told me, "I personally don't record lectures because few of my classes are lecture-based." In other words, her discussion-based and small-group classes don't lend themselves to a recorded format. However, she works hard to create an accessible course by providing extensive accessibility options for her students: "I have a Zoom option for live attendance for students who can't attend in person. I provide detailed notes that I take during class via Google Docs. Finally, I provide a slide deck if I use one. And to accompany all of this, I have a flexible attendance policy." If you cannot share your class recordings, there are many other methods to ensure that mentally disabled students have ways to access similar information. And remember, only sharing your recordings is not enough to have an accessible course.

Do Not Invade Students' Privacy for Accommodations

If you have been teaching for a while, you have likely had at least one student request disability accommodations. Typical accommodations include extra time on exams, a quiet room in which to take an exam, or special seating in a classroom. Think about how you treat a student who approaches you with an accommodation request. Are you kind and welcoming? Neutral? Aggravated that your smooth-running class is interrupted by a student's need for something extra?

Fear of disability fakers—fear of "the disability con," as disability legal studies scholar Doron Dorfman puts it—is pervasive in US culture.[28] The belief that people fake disabilities to get special rights or privileges is an element of ableism, and we all suffer from internalized ableism. If a student comes to you asking for learning accommodations, and you feel that pinch of doubt that tells you the student is faking, stop yourself. If you think, "How can every student have ADHD? It's so overdiagnosed." Stop. Just stop.

If you are concerned about students having extra time on your exams, create exams that do not need a time limit to accurately test student learning. (Yes, really.) Ask yourself whether your course is supposed to be assessing speediness. Literally: Is speediness one of your course goals? If so, are you teaching speediness to your students? Except in rare cases, the answer to these questions is no. And if the answer is no, a time limit on your exam is an unnecessary logistical hurdle for your students. I know firsthand what a speediness course goal looks like—I teach a course in which students must write legal documents in a 90-minute period to prepare for the bar exam. In this course, speediness is a course goal on the syllabus, a component of my teaching, and an outcome that I assess. Let's give ourselves space to rethink time limits on exams.

Rather than being suspicious of your students who request accommodations, be grateful that you have the opportunity to teach a diverse group of students and include them in your course in ways that can help them succeed. Go a step further than their accommodation and collaborate with them; ask if there is anything more that you can do to help them succeed. The best part is that you learn ways to make your teaching better for all of your students.

When a student comes to you to request an accommodation, do you ever ask the student what their disability is? You should never do this. The information is confidential, legally. But as a professor, you have great influence over your students, so your student will likely tell you even if doing so makes them uncomfortable. As disability legal studies scholar Katherine Macfarlane explains, "When students are required to deliver accommodation letters to their professors, those professors may force a conversation about the accommodations and require students to disclose more than the content of the letters."[29] Asking that students share their private information is infantilizing. Instead of acting suspicious or invading their privacy, treat disabled students who approach you for accommodations with respect and kindness. Thank them for sharing their accommodation needs with you—after all, you want all of your students to have the opportunity to do well in your class. (Right?) If you are struggling to have a positive attitude about accommodations, examine your own thought processes to discover whether you feel skeptical of disabled students—and eradicate that element of ableism from your brain.

We must remember that our students are adults. Whether you teach college freshmen (like I did for a decade) or third-year law students (like I do now), you are teaching grown-ups. They sometimes make immature decisions, or just plain bad decisions. But rather than allowing those bad decisions to drive us to clamp down on their autonomy, we must remember that our students are noble, courageous, and full of generous ideas. So yes, our students will make mistakes, but our job as their professors is to help them learn from those mistakes, not punish them. Punitive pedagogy only puts a student who has made a mistake deeper into the hole they are already in.

I am asking all of us to open our minds about how good learning happens. We agree that we want our students to learn as much as possible. We have common ground. But then, unfortunately, some of us diverge. There are rigor angsters at one end of the spectrum, and those who teach accessibly/inclusively at the other. In the middle are those who borrow some teaching ideas from both.

Instead, let us fully embrace accessible/inclusive teaching to help students learn how to cultivate their own internal success tools. You cannot hammer students into shape like a metalsmith. They will only learn that learning hurts, that it is punitive and something to fear. We must help our students feel empowered. When a person feels empowered, they are open to new ideas. For some professors, empowering students means letting go of the idea that students must be forced to learn and instead believing that they want to learn. I believe that students want to learn. Join me.

Acknowledgments

This book has been six years in the making. Ever since *Life of the Mind Interrupted* came out in 2017, I knew I wanted to write another book on mental disability in higher education. But so much had changed since 2017. I went from being a mother of elementary-aged children to the mother of teens; I was (formally) diagnosed with autism; my relationship with academia waned and then waxed again (to my surprise). With all of these changes, I knew this book would be very different from the first one. Worse, despite my love of this topic and eagerness to write about it, I feared that this book would not live up to its predecessor or do the important work that I needed it to do.

When I mentioned this fear about my writing to my friend and colleague Karen Ray Costa, she wrote this reply (lightly edited): "There is an immense amount of pressure on those of us writing from various marginalized spaces to be perfect, and it's too much. So I focus on doing my part, interdependence, and improving upon the pile of crap we have now." So here is this book, where I do my part, rely on others immensely and allow them to rely on me, and hopefully make the world better.

Fortunately, I have had a team of supporters making sure that this book is as good as it could possibly be. They deserve a large share of credit for the book's strengths; its flaws are my own.

I would like to thank my earliest readers, who gave me valuable feedback on the manuscript and proposal before I ever submitted it for consideration: Janie Chang, Alexa Z. Chew, Lauren Faulkenberry, Rachel Selinger, and Camille Pagán.

A very special thanks to my new writing group, who dropped into my life at just the right time and walked with me through the drafting and revising of this book: Bronwyn Charlton and Ayla Samli (and Erin

McElligott, if only for a short while). I am so pleased that we found each other. I *absolutely* could not have written this book without you.

Another special thanks to my final readers, all of whom are excellent writers and most of whom are good friends, who read the manuscript in part or in its entirety—an enormous task—before I submitted it to the publisher: Kelly J. Baker, Emily Colin, Elizabeth Donaldson, Teresa Heinz Housel, and Jordynn Jack.

Thanks to my editors at the *Chronicle of Higher Education*, where some of these ideas were first explored, Denise Magner and Jess Engebretson. Thanks also to my editor at the *Journal of the Legal Writing Institute*, Wayne Scheiss, for the same reason.

Thanks to the Junior (Justice) League Publishing Committee, Kelly Harms and Camille Pagán, for encouraging me to hold fast to my vision for both this book and my publishing career. Friends, it doesn't matter how we came together; it only matters that we did.

Thanks to my friend, colleague, and so much more Alexa Z. Chew, who held my hand with this project from start to finish, and who does so all the time.

Thank you to my UNC Law students whom I taught while I wrote this book; because of FERPA, I am not going to name you here, except for Nolon, because you gave me permission. To those students whose words I quoted throughout this book, thank you for speaking the truth out loud. It is never easy to do so, especially when you are at the beginning of your career. You are leaders, and you will do amazing things.

I would like to thank all of the people who have read and supported my writing on mental disability in the past, in particular my book *Life of the Mind Interrupted*. Your support inspired me to write this book, and it kept me going when the writing got really, really hard. (And boy, it got really hard there for a while.) I would like to include special thanks to institutions that brought me in to speak on mental health over the years, including Hope College, Macalester College, Johnson County Community College, and West Chester University. Thank you for letting me share my ideas on disability, accessibility, and inclusivity with students and faculty around the country. Your communities inspire me. Thank you to my agents, Tom and Luke Neilssen, and BrightSight Speakers for helping me reach others beyond my small town of Chapel Hill.

I would like to thank my disability and pedagogy colleagues and friends, who are too many to name, but I will try, and in no order of importance, but alphabetically:

Alice Wong,
Ann Gagné,
Cait Gordon,
Cate Denial,
Catherine Prendergast,
Claire McGuire,
The Cyborg Jillian Weise,
Danielle Tully,
Doron Dorfman,
Ellie Margolis,
Farrell Jenab,
Grace Lapointe,
Jordynn Jack,
Karrie Higgins,
Kat Macfarlane,
Kathy Flaherty,

Keith J. Myers,
Kelly J. Baker,
Kevin Gannon,
Kevin McClure,
Lauren Cagle,
Lee Skallerup-Bessette,
Margaret Price,
Martha Crawford,
Nyasha Junior,
Porochista Khakpour,
Rebecca Pope-Ruark,
Rick Godden,
Sarah J. Schendel,
Sean Michael Morris,
Viji Sathy,
and so many more.

If I forgot to mention you, I sincerely apologize—you are in my heart.

I would like to thank my ever-supportive colleagues at the University of North Carolina School of Law, including Alexa Z. Chew, Rachel Gurvich, Sara Warf, Kaci Bishop, Kevin Bennardo, Pete Nemerovski, Craig Smith, Leigh Osofsky, O. J. Salinas, Luke Everett, and Annie Scardulla. Thank you for your constant support of my research and writing.

Thank you to my entire team at the University Press of Kansas: my editor David Congdon, Stephanie Marshall Ward, Kelly Chrisman Jacques, Derek Helms, Karl Janssen, Suzanne Galle, and Alec Loganbill.

Thanks to my early publishers Blue Crow Books (print) and Blackstone (audio), who published *Life of the Mind Interrupted*. You (we) made this new book possible.

Closer to home, I would like to thank Annie Johnston and her spaces La Vita Dolce and Market & Moss. Annie is my friend, and she provides my place to write and my place to celebrate. (Thanks to you too, Erin P-F, even as you take your journey elsewhere.)

And finally, thank you to my family:

Thanks to my parents, who, over the years, were never quite sure what to do with a writer in the family, but who have always bought my books, read my books, come to my book launches, and made their friends do the same. This apple might have fallen far from the tree, but the tree is big and giving.

Thanks to my Aunt C., who spent years teaching my children, and also me.

Thanks to my sister Chris, who has always been my best friend, my walkie-talkie, and my biggest fan—now my neighbor, *thank goodness*, since Mr. Rogers did *not* prepare us for this. And thank you to the rest of her family—my little bro, and my sobrino and sobrinas. I love you all.

Thanks to Michael, my spouse and partner in all things, who supports and believes in me and never makes me feel wrong or weird, who sat in a dark car one night in 2009 and listened to me tell him that I have bipolar disorder and said, "Okay," and I said, "No, really, it's bad" and started crying, and he said we'd figure it out—and we did, and here we are. I love you.

Thank you to my sparkling sprites, 14 and 12, who inspire me more than anything else in the world. How could you not? You glow like stars. You are immense.

Notes

PREFACE

1. Marc Bousquet, "The Rhetoric of 'Job Market' and the Reality of the Academic Labor System," *College English* 66, no. 2 (November 2003): 207–228, https://doi.org/10.2307/3594266.

2. Katie Rose Guest Pryal, "Front-Line Faculty and Systemic Burnout: Why More Faculty Should Attend to Law Students' Mental Health and the Inequities Caused by Faculty Who Opt Out," *Legal Writing: The Journal of the Legal Writing Institute* 27, no. 1 (2023): 199–221.

3. Katie J. M. Baker, "How Colleges Flunk Mental Health," *Newsweek*, February 11, 2014, https://perma.cc/V4JD-47ML, https://www.newsweek.com/2014/02/14/how-colleges-flunk-mental-health-245492.html.

4. Kasey Meeks, Amy Sutton Peak, and Adam Dreihaus, "Depression, Anxiety, and Stress among Students, Faculty, and Staff," *Journal of American College Health* 71, no. 2 (February 12, 2023): 348–354, https://doi.org/10.1080/07448481.2021.1891913.

5. National Institute of Mental Health, "Any Anxiety Disorder," *National Institute of Mental Health*, accessed March 23, 2023, https://www.nimh.nih.gov/health/statistics/any-anxiety-disorder.

6. Katie Rose Guest Pryal, *Life of the Mind Interrupted: Essays on Mental Health and Disability in Higher Education* (Chapel Hill, NC: Blue Crow Books, 2017), xv.

7. Pryal, *Life of the Mind Interrupted*, 8.

8. Margaret Price, *Mad at School: Rhetorics of Mental Disability and Academic Life* (Ann Arbor: University of Michigan Press, 2011), 6.

9. M. Remi Yergeau, "Clinically Significant Disturbance: On Theorists Who Theorize Theory of Mind," *Disability Studies Quarterly* 33, no. 4 (September 5, 2013), https://doi.org/10.18061/dsq.v33i4.3876.

10. Karen Ray Costa, "Is COVID a Collective Trauma?" *Karen Ray Costa*, February 9, 2022, https://karenraycosta.medium.com/is-covid-a-collective-trauma-e83bb1c2e2a7.

11. Karen Ray Costa, "The Next Phase," *Karen Ray Costa*, May 19, 2021, https://karenraycosta.medium.com/the-next-phase-a7912bc6a453.

12. Joseph Fruscione and Kelly J. Baker, "Introduction," in *Succeeding Outside the Academy: Career Paths beyond the Humanities, Social Sciences, and STEM*, ed. Joseph Fruscione and Kelly J. Baker (Lawrence: University Press of Kansas, 2018), 2.

13. Rachel López, "Unentitled: The Power of Designation in the Legal Academy," *Rutgers University Law Review* 73, no. 3 (Spring 2021): 923–932.

14. Kate Kaul, "Risking Experience: Disability, Precarity, and Disclosure," in *Negotiating Disability: Disclosure and Higher Education*, ed. Stephanie L. Kerschbaum, Laura T. Eisenman, and James M. Jones (Ann Arbor: University of Michigan Press, 2017), 171–187, https://doi.org/10.3998/mpub.9426902.

INTRODUCTION

1. Andy Meek, "NRA's Wayne LaPierre: 'Good Guys with Guns' Could Have Stopped Navy Yard Shooting," *Time*, September 22, 2013, http://nation.time .com/2013/09/22/nras-wayne-lapierre-good-guys-with-guns-could-have -stopped-navy-yard-shooting/. See also Katie Rose Guest Pryal, "Heller's Scapegoats," *North Carolina Law Review* 93, no. 5 (June 2015): 1439–1474.

2. Thomas Lu and Sylvie Douglis, "Don't Be Scared to Talk about Disabilities: Here's What to Know and What to Say," *NPR*, February 22, 2022, https:// perma.cc/D5KU-A8C3, https://www.npr.org/2022/02/18/1081713756/disability -disabled-people-offensive-better-word.

3. American Psychiatric Association, "What Is Mental Illness?" *American Psychiatric Association*, https://perma.cc/B47X-3K6N, accessed March 24, 2023, https://psychiatry.org/patients-families/what-is-mental-illness.

4. Price, *Mad at School*, 12.

5. Andrew Solomon, *The Noonday Demon: An Atlas of Depression* (New York: Scribner, 2001), 79.

6. Centers for Disease Control and Prevention, "Facts about Developmental Disabilities," *CDC*, https://perma.cc/5MK4-TWKC, accessed March 23, 2023, https://www.cdc.gov/ncbddd/developmentaldisabilities/facts.html.

7. Centers for Disease Control and Prevention, "What Is Autism Spectrum Disorder," *CDC*, https://perma.cc/PKV6-2U7H, accessed March 23, 2023, https://www.cdc.gov/ncbddd/autism/facts.html.

8. Evan DeVries and The Thompson Policy Institute, "Comparing Mental Illness and Intellectual and Developmental Disabilities," *Chapman University*, August 2, 2016, https://blogs.chapman.edu/tpi/2016/08/02/comparing-men tal-illness-and-intellectual-and-developmental-disabilities/.

9. Giulia Perini et al., "Cognitive Impairment in Depression: Recent Advances and Novel Treatments," *Neuropsychiatric Disease and Treatment* 15 (May 2019): 1250, https://doi.org/10.2147/NDT.S199746.

10. Nelson Cowan, "Working Memory Underpins Cognitive Development, Learning, and Education," *Educational Psychology Review* 26, no. 2 (June 1, 2014): 197, https://doi.org/10.1007/s10648-013-9246-y.

11. Suneeta Kercood et al., "Working Memory and Autism: A Review of Literature," *Research in Autism Spectrum Disorders* 8, no. 10 (October 1, 2014): 1316–1332, https://doi.org/10.1016/j.rasd.2014.06.011.

12. Cleveland Clinic, "Neurodivergent," *Cleveland Clinic*, accessed April 1, 2023, https://my.clevelandclinic.org/health/symptoms/23154-neurodivergent.

13. Judy Singer, "'Why Can't You Be Normal for Once in Your Life?': From a 'Problem with No Name' to the Emergence of a New Category of Difference," in *Disability Discourse*, ed. Mairian Corker and Sally French (Philadelphia: Open University Press, 1999), 64. Singer coined the term in her 1998 honors thesis at the University of Technology in Sydney, Australia, before publishing this book chapter.

14. For example, see Matthew P. Janicki, James A. Hendrix, and Philip Mc-Callion, "Examining Older Adults with Neuroatypical Conditions for MCI/Dementia: Barriers and Recommendations of the Neuroatypical Conditions Expert Consultative Panel," *Alzheimer's & Dementia : Diagnosis, Assessment & Disease Monitoring* 14, no. 1 (July 8, 2022): e12335, https://doi.org/10.1002/dad2.12335.

15. Price, *Mad at School*, 19. Price gives credit to disability studies scholar Cynthia Lewiecki-Wilson for the phrase.

16. Ashe Grey, "Bad Crip: A Probably Not Comprehensive Definition," *Crippled Scholar*, March 14, 2016, https://perma.cc/6N9Q-SU8G, https://crippled-scholar.com/2016/03/14/bad-crip-a-probably-not-comprehensive-definition/.

17. Rosemarie Garland-Thomson, *Extraordinary Bodies: Figuring Physical Disability in American Culture and Literature* (New York: Columbia University Press, 2017), 8.

18. Rosemarie Garland-Thomson, *Staring: How We Look* (New York: Oxford University Press, 2009), 202 (note 19 to chapter 4).

19. Lydia X. Z. Brown, "Ableism/Language," *Autistic Hoya*, September 14, 2022, http://autistichoya.com/ableist-words-and-terms-to-avoid.html.

20. Price, *Mad at School*, 8.

21. Bruce G. Link and Jo C. Phelan, "Conceptualizing Stigma," *Annual Review of Sociology* 27, no. 1 (August 2001): 367, https://doi.org/10.1146/annurev.soc.27.1.363.

22. Amy F. Crocker and Susan N. Smith, "Person-First Language: Are We Practicing What We Preach?" *Journal of Multidisciplinary Healthcare* 12 (February 8, 2019): 125–129, https://doi.org/10.2147/JMDH.S140067.

23. Lydia X. Z. Brown, "Identity-First Language," *Autistic Self Advocacy Network*, March 2, 2012, https://perma.cc/5L6C-7SDM, https://autisticadvocacy.org/about-asan/identity-first-language/.

24. Doron Dorfman, "[Un]Usual Suspects: Deservingness, Scarcity, and

Disability Rights," *University of California at Irvine Law Review* 10, no. 2 (2020): 564.

25. Hannah Belcher, "Autistic People and Masking," *National Autistic Society (UK)*, July 7, 2022, https://perma.cc/68PT-E2N2, https://www.autism.org.uk/advice-and-guidance/professional-practice/autistic-masking.

26. Laura Hull et al., "'Putting on My Best Normal': Social Camouflaging in Adults with Autism Spectrum Conditions," *Journal of Autism and Developmental Disorders* 47, no. 8 (August 2017): 2521, https://doi.org/10.1007/s10803-017-3166-5.

27. Doron Dorfman, "Fear of the Disability Con: Perceptions of Fraud and Special Rights Discourse," *Law and Society Review* 53, no. 4 (December 2019): 1060, https://doi.org/10.1111/lasr.12437.

28. Dorfman, "Fear of the Disability Con," 1053.

29. Pryal, *Life of the Mind Interrupted*, 102.

30. Jennifer C. Sarrett, "Autism and Accommodations in Higher Education: Insights from the Autism Community," *Journal of Autism and Developmental Disorders* 48, no. 3 (March 2018): 685, https://doi.org/10.1007/s10803-017-3353-4.

31. Pryal, L*ife of the Mind Interrupted*, 103.

CHAPTER 1. ANXIETY IN ACADEMIA

1. Joseph A. Kim et al., "The Prevalence of Anxiety and Mood Problems among Children with Autism and Asperger Syndrome," *Autism* 4, no. 2 (June 1, 2000): 117–132.

2. Kasey Meeks, Amy Sutton Peak, and Adam Dreihaus, "Depression, Anxiety, and Stress among Students, Faculty, and Staff," *Journal of American College Health* 71, no. 2 (February 12, 2023): 348–354.

3. National Institute of Mental Health, "Any Anxiety Disorder," *NIMH*, accessed March 23, 2023, https://www.nimh.nih.gov/health/statistics/any-anxiety-disorder.

4. Claire Bond Potter, "The Hard Truths of the Academic-Labor Crisis," *Chronicle of Higher Education*, November 17, 2022, https://www.chronicle.com/article/the-hard-truths-of-the-academic-labor-crisis.

5. Potter, "The Hard Truths of the Academic-Labor Crisis."

6. Gretchen M. Reevy and Grace Deason, "Predictors of Depression, Stress, and Anxiety among Non-Tenure Track Faculty," *Frontiers in Psychology* 5, no. 701 (July 8, 2014): 1–17.

7. Owen Kelly, "What Are Anxiety Disorders?" *Verywell Mind*, May 14, 2022, https://perma.cc/RXB2-ZVZC, https://www.verywellmind.com/anxiety-disorder-2510539.

8. American Psychiatric Association, "Generalized Anxiety Disorder," in

Diagnostic and Statistical Manual of Mental Disorders, 5th-TR, online ed. (Washington, DC: APA Publishing, 2022), https://dsm.psychiatryonline.org /doi/book/10.1176/appi.books.9780890425787.

9. American Psychiatric Association, "Generalized Anxiety Disorder."

10. Interview, April 13, 2023, via email.

11. Graham C. L. Davey and Suzannah Levy, "Catastrophic Worrying: Personal Inadequacy and a Perseverative Iterative Style as Features of the Catastrophizing Process," *Journal of Abnormal Psychology* 107 (1998): 576.

12. Susan Nolen-Hoeksema, Blair E. Wisco, and Sonja Lyubomirsky, "Rethinking Rumination," *Perspectives on Psychological Science* 3, no. 5 (September 2008): 400.

13. Kendra Cherry, "What Is the Illusion of Control?" *Verywell Mind*, August 3, 2022, https://perma.cc/K39T-M2CC, https://www.verywellmind.com /what-is-the-illusion-of-control-5198406.

14. Nolen-Hoeksema, Wisco, and Lyubomirsky, "Rethinking Rumination," 400.

15. Devon Price, "Laziness Does Not Exist," *Human Parts*, March 23, 2018, https://perma.cc/LZ8J-LXWU, https://humanparts.medium.com/laziness-does -not-exist-3af27e312d01. See also: Devon Price, *Laziness Does Not Exist: A Defense of the Exhausted, Exploited, and Overworked* (New York: Simon and Schuster, 2021).

16. Alison L. Flett, Mohsen Haghbin, and Timothy A. Pychyl, "Procrastination and Depression from a Cognitive Perspective: An Exploration of the Associations among Procrastinatory Automatic Thoughts, Rumination, and Mindfulness," *Journal of Rational-Emotive & Cognitive-Behavior Therapy* 34, no. 3 (September 2016): 169–186.

CHAPTER 2. POPULATION SHOCK EVENTS

1. COVID-19 Mental Disorders Collaborators, "Global Prevalence and Burden of Depressive and Anxiety Disorders in 204 Countries and Territories in 2020 Due to the COVID-19 Pandemic," *The Lancet* 398, no. 10312 (November 2021): 1708.

2. Note that in the field of economics, the term "population shock" has a different meaning, describing a large change in the number of people in a region. See, for example, Abel Schumann, "Persistence of Population Shocks: Evidence from the Occupation of West Germany after World War II," *American Economic Journal: Applied Economics* 6, no. 3 (July 2014): 189–205.

3. COVID-19 Mental Disorders Collaborators, "Global Prevalence and Burden of Depressive and Anxiety Disorders," 1708.

4. Emerson College Emergency Management, "ALICE Training," *Emerson College*, https://perma.cc/CV28-EEHB, accessed January 1, 2023, https://

emerson.edu/departments/emergency-management/safety-awareness-train
ings/alice-training.

5. See, for example, this discussion of lifelike drills for K–12 students covered by Rachel M. Cohen, "Are Active Shooter Drills Worth It?" *Vox*, May 28, 2022, https://perma.cc/8NQN-FZVZ, https://www.vox.com/23144105/lockdown-drills
-active-shooter-uvalde-robb-texas.

6. Joshua Gordon, "One Year In: COVID-19 and Mental Health," *National Institute of Mental Health (NIMH)*, April 9, 2021, https://perma.cc/TYL3
-M5F2, https://www.nimh.nih.gov/about/director/messages/2021/one-year-in
-covid-19-and-mental-health.

7. Mark É. Czeisler et al., "Mental Health, Substance Use, and Suicidal Ideation during the COVID-19 Pandemic—United States, June 24–30, 2020," *Centers for Disease Control Morbidity and Mortality Weekly Report* 69, no. 32 (August 14, 2020): 1049–1057.

8. COVID-19 Mental Disorders Collaborators, "Global Prevalence and Burden of Depressive and Anxiety Disorders," 1708.

9. Gilad Hirschberger, "Collective Trauma and the Social Construction of Meaning," *Frontiers in Psychology* 9 (August 10, 2018): 1441.

10. Hirschberger, "Collective Trauma and the Social Construction of Meaning."

11. Karen Ray Costa, "Is COVID a Collective Trauma?" *Karen Ray Costa*, February 9, 2022, https://perma.cc/2YMH-5Y2Z, https://karenraycosta.medium
.com/is-covid-a-collective-trauma-e83bb1c2e2a7.

12. Interview, September 2022, in-person, Chapel Hill, NC.

13. Costa, "Is COVID a Collective Trauma?"

14. Gabriele Ciciurkaite, Guadalupe Marquez-Velarde, and Robyn Lewis Brown, "Stressors Associated with the COVID-19 Pandemic, Disability, and Mental Health: Considerations from the Intermountain West," *Stress and Health* 38, no. 2 (April 2022): 305.

15. Bridget M. Kuehn, "Clinician Shortage Exacerbates Pandemic-Fueled 'Mental Health Crisis,'" *JAMA* 327, no. 22 (June 14, 2022): 2179.

16. Alice Wong, *Year of the Tiger: An Activist's Life* (New York: Vintage, 2022), 337.

17. Costa, "Is COVID a Collective Trauma?"

CHAPTER 3. SYSTEMIC BURNOUT

1. Rebecca Pope-Ruark, *Unraveling Faculty Burnout: Pathways to Reckoning and Renewal* (Baltimore: Johns Hopkins University Press, 2022), 7.

2. World Health Organization News, "Burn-Out an 'Occupational Phenomenon': International Classification of Diseases," *World Health Organization*, May 28, 2019, https://www.who.int/news/item/28-05-2019-burn-out
-an-occupational-phenomenon-international-classification-of-diseases.

3. Christina Maslach, Wilmar B. Schaufeli, and Michael P. Leiter, "Job Burnout," *Annual Review of Psychology* 52, no. 1 (February 2001): 399.

4. Maslach, Schaufeli, and Leiter, "Job Burnout," 398.

5. Joseph Fruscione and Kelly J. Baker, "Introduction," in *Succeeding Outside the Academy: Career Paths beyond the Humanities, Social Sciences, and STEM*, ed. Joseph Fruscione and Kelly J. Baker (Lawrence: University Press of Kansas, 2018), 2.

6. Gretchen M. Reevy and Grace Deason, "Predictors of Depression, Stress, and Anxiety among Non-Tenure Track Faculty," *Frontiers in Psychology* 5 (July 8, 2014), 1.

7. Reevy and Deason, "Predictors of Depression," 13.

8. Pope-Ruark, *Unraveling Faculty Burnout*, 9.

9. Kristen R. Choi et al., "A Second Pandemic: Mental Health Spillover from the Novel Coronavirus (COVID-19)," *Journal of the American Psychiatric Nurses Association* 26, no. 4 (July 2020): 340–343.

10. Sherrill W. Hayes et al., "Perceived Stress, Work-Related Burnout, and Working from Home before and during COVID-19: An Examination of Workers in the United States," *SAGE Open* 11, no. 4 (October 2021): 3.

11. Pope-Ruark, *Unraveling Faculty Burnout*, 12.

12. Kevin R. McClure, "Don't Blame the Pandemic for Worker Discontent," *Chronicle of Higher Education*, May 27, 2022, https://www.chronicle.com/arti cle/dont-blame-the-pandemic-for-worker-discontent.

13. Kevin R. McClure and Alisa Hicklin Fryar, "The Great Faculty Disengagement," *Chronicle of Higher Education*, January 19, 2022, https://perma.cc /QXP5-GKJH, https://www.chronicle.com/article/the-great-faculty-disengage ment.

14. UNC Human Resources and Equal Opportunity and Compliance, "Wellness," University of North Carolina at Chapel Hill, https://perma.cc/578W -SPZM, accessed October 1, 2022, https://hr.unc.edu/return-to-campus/well ness/.

15. Pope-Ruark, *Unraveling Faculty Burnout*, 21.

16. Katie Rose Guest Pryal, "Disclosure Blues: Should You Tell Colleagues about Your Mental Illness?" *Chronicle of Higher Education*, June 13, 2014.

CHAPTER 4. TOXIC ACADEMIC OVERWORK

1. Marc Bousquet, "The Rhetoric of 'Job Market' and the Reality of the Academic Labor System," *College English* 66, no. 2 (November 2003): 221.

2. Anton Muscatelli, "Universities Must Overhaul the Toxic Working Culture for Academic Researchers," *The Guardian*, January 15, 2020, https://perma.cc /MM58-Y87N, https://www.theguardian.com/education/2020/jan/15/universi ties-must-overhaul-the-toxic-working-culture-for-academic-researchers.

3. Maria LaMonaca Wisdom, "What Is the Real Cost of Academe's Fixation

on Productivity?" *Chronicle of Higher Education*, May 5, 2022, https://www
.chronicle.com/article/what-is-the-real-cost-of-academes-fixation-on-produc
tivity.

4. Rebecca Pope-Ruark, *Unraveling Faculty Burnout: Pathways to Reckoning and Renewal* (Baltimore: Johns Hopkins University Press, 2022), 26.

5. Pope-Ruark, *Unraveling Faculty Burnout*, 26.

6. Hilal A. Lashuel, "Mental Health in Academia: What about Faculty?"
ELife 9 (January 8, 2020): e54551.

7. Kaci Bishop, "Framing Failure in the Legal Classroom: Techniques for Encouraging Growth and Resilience," *Arkansas Law Review* 70, no. 4 (2018): 960.

8. Kasey Meeks, Amy Sutton Peak, and Adam Dreihaus, "Depression, Anxiety, and Stress among Students, Faculty, and Staff," *Journal of American College
Health* 71, no. 2 (February 12, 2023): 348–354.

9. Lashuel, "What About Faculty?"

10. Lashuel, "What About Faculty?"

11. Margaret Price, *Mad at School, Rhetorics of Mental Disability and Academic Life* (Ann Arbor: University of Michigan Press, 2011), 33.

12. Pope-Ruark, *Unraveling Faculty Burnout*, 26.

13. Kevin R. McClure, "Don't Blame the Pandemic for Worker Discontent,"
Chronicle of Higher Education, May 27, 2022, https://www.chronicle.com/arti
cle/dont-blame-the-pandemic-for-worker-discontent.

14. McClure, "Don't Blame the Pandemic."

15. Pope-Ruark, *Unraveling Faculty Burnout*, 7.

CHAPTER 5. SETTING BOUNDARIES

1. Anne Katherine, "Create Boundaries," *Your Cherished Life*, https://perma
.cc/A6PW-LK2B, accessed October 6, 2022, https://1annekatherine.com/http
wp-mep39g1w-z/. See also, Anne Katherine, *Where to Draw the Line: How to Set
Healthy Boundaries Every Day* (New York: Touchstone, 2012).

2. Meera E. Deo, "Pandemic Pressures on Faculty," *University of Pennsylvania Law Review Online* 170, no. 1 (2022): 131, https://scholarship.law.upenn
.edu/penn_law_review_online/vol170/iss1/8/.

3. Cassandra M. Guarino and Victor M. H. Borden, "Faculty Service Loads
and Gender: Are Women Taking Care of the Academic Family," *Research in
Higher Education* 58, no. 6 (September 1, 2017): 672. See also, Kelly J. Baker,
Sexism Ed: Essays on Gender and Labor in Academia (Chapel Hill, NC: Blue
Crow Books, 2018).

4. Renee Nicole Allen, Alicia Jackson, and DeShun Harris, "The 'Pink Ghetto'
Pipeline: Challenges and Opportunities for Women in Legal Education," *University of Detroit Mercy Law Review* 96, no. 2 (Summer 2019): 525–555.

5. Debra A. Harley, "Maids of Academe: African American Women Faculty

at Predominately White Institutions," *Journal of African American Studies* 12, no. 1 (2008): 19.

6. Amado M. Padilla, "Ethnic Minority Scholars, Research, and Mentoring: Current and Future Issues," *Educational Researcher* 23, no. 4 (May 1994): 26.

7. Padilla, "Ethnic Minority Scholars," 26.

8. Padilla, "Ethnic Minority Scholars," 26.

9. Taleed El-Sabawi and Madison Fields, eds., "The Discounted Labor of BI-POC Students & Faculty," *California Law Review Online* 12, no. 1212849 (2021): 24.

10. El-Sabawi and Fields, "The Discounted Labor of BIPOC Students & Faculty," 24.

11. National Center for Education Statistics, "A Majority of College Students with Disabilities Do Not Inform School, New NCES Data Show," *National Center for Education Statistics*, April 26, 2022, https://nces.ed.gov/whatsnew/press_releases/4_26_2022.asp; Margaret Price et al., "Disclosure of Mental Disability by College and University Faculty: The Negotiation of Accommodations, Supports, and Barriers," *Disability Studies Quarterly* 37, no. 2 (June 1, 2017).

12. Katherine Macfarlane, "Disability without Documentation," *Fordham Law Review* 90, no. 1 (2021): 70.

13. Katie Rose Guest Pryal, *Life of the Mind Interrupted: Essays on Mental Health and Disability in Higher Education* (Chapel Hill, NC: Blue Crow Books, 2017), 53.

14. Sarah J. Schendel, "Due Dates in the Real World: Extensions, Equity, and the Hidden Curriculum," *Georgetown Journal of Legal Ethics* 35, no. 2 (2022): 207.

15. Melissa Febos, "Do You Want to Be Known for Your Writing, or for Your Swift Email Responses?" *Catapult*, March 23, 2017, https://perma.cc/V6ES-B93G, https://catapult.co/stories/do-you-want-to-be-known-for-your-writing-or-for-your-swift-email-responses.

CHAPTER 6. THE DISABLED MIND IN ACADEMIA

1. Bruce G. Link et al., "Public Conceptions of Mental Illness: Labels, Causes, Dangerousness, and Social Distance," *American Journal of Public Health* 89, no. 9 (September 1999): 1328–1333.

2. Katherine Anne Comtois, "A Review of Interventions to Reduce the Prevalence of Parasuicide," *Psychiatric Services* 53, no. 9 (September 2002): 1138.

3. Nicholas A. Hubbard et al., "Depressive Thoughts Limit Working Memory Capacity in Dysphoria," *Cognition and Emotion* 30, no. 2 (February 17, 2016): 206.

4. Link et al., "Public Conceptions of Mental Illness."

5. Lennard Davis, "Introduction," in *Disability Studies Reader*, 2nd ed., ed. Lennard Davis (New York: Routledge, 1997), xv.

6. Clara Bergen et al., "Communication in Youth Mental Health Clinical Encounters: Introducing the Agential Stance," *Theory and Psychology* 32, no. 5 (October 2022): 669.

7. Catherine Prendergast, "On the Rhetorics of Mental Disability," in *Embodied Rhetorics: Disability in Language and Culture*, ed. James C. Wilson and Cynthia Lewiecki-Wilson (Carbondale: Southern Illinois University Press, 2003), 203.

8. Corbett O'Toole, "Disclosing Our Relationships to Disabilities: An Invitation for Disability Studies Scholars," *Disability Studies Quarterly* 33, no. 2 (March 27, 2013).

9. Kate Kaul, "Risking Experience: Disability, Precarity, and Disclosure," in *Negotiating Disability: Disclosure and Higher Education*, ed. Stephanie L. Kerschbaum, Laura T. Eisenman, and James M. Jones (Ann Arbor: University of Michigan Press, 2017), 171–187.

10. Kaul, "Risking Experience," 177.

11. Joseph Fruscione and Kelly J. Baker, "Introduction," in *Succeeding Outside the Academy: Career Paths beyond the Humanities, Social Sciences, and STEM*, ed. Joseph Fruscione and Kelly J. Baker (Lawrence: University Press of Kansas, 2018), 3.

12. Kaul, "Risking Experience," 183.

13. Kaul, "Risking Experience," 178.

14. Katie Rose Guest Pryal, "How the TSA Perpetuates Harmful Mental Health Stigmas," *The Establishment*, May 12, 2016, https://perma.cc/7E2J-78SC, https://medium.com/the-establishment/how-the-tsa-perpetuates-harmful-mental-health-stigmas-90f531962158.

CHAPTER 7. WRITING PUBLICLY ABOUT MENTAL DISABILITY

1. Anna Chang, "MLA Publishes New Guidelines on Evaluating Publicly Engaged Humanities Scholarship," *MLA Commons*, August 17, 2022, https://perma.cc/PPP9-87B3, https://news.mla.hcommons.org/2022/08/17/mla-publishes-new-guidelines-on-evaluating-publicly-engaged-humanities-scholarship/.

2. See Katie Rose Guest Pryal, "How to Write Publicly about Rape," in *Even If You're Broken: Essays on Sexual Assault and #MeToo* by Katie Rose Guest Pryal (Chapel Hill, NC: Blue Crow Books, 2019).

3. Doron Dorfman, "Fear of the Disability Con: Perceptions of Fraud and Special Rights Discourse," *Law and Society Review* 53, no. 4 (December 2019): 1051–1091.

4. Katie Rose Guest Pryal, "My Disability Story Isn't for Your Catharsis," *The*

Establishment, September 25, 2018, https://perma.cc/V7Z8-6UGR, https://theestablishment.co/my-disability-story-isnt-for-your-catharsis/index.html.

5. Katie Rose Guest Pryal, *Life of the Mind Interrupted: Essays on Mental Health and Disability in Higher Education* (Chapel Hill, NC: Blue Crow Books, 2017).

6. See, for example, Katie Rose Guest Pryal, "The World Doesn't Bend for Disabled Kids (or Disabled Parents)," *Catapult*, July 10, 2018, https://perma.cc/ZX2L-JX9E, https://catapult.co/stories/the-world-doesnt-bend-for-disabled-kids-or-disabled-parents.

7. Tressie McMillan Cottom, "'Who Do You Think You Are?': When Marginality Meets Academic Microcelebrity," *Ada: A Journal of Gender, New Media, and Technology* 7 (2015), https://doi.org/10.7264/N3319T5T.

8. Tressie McMillan Cottom, "Everything but the Burden: Publics, Public Scholarship, and Institutions," *Some of Us Are Brave: The Archive*, May 12, 2015, https://perma.cc/2MUQ-DZYY, https://tressiemc.com/uncategorized/everything-but-the-burden-publics-public-scholarship-and-institutions/.

9. Kelly J. Baker, "Crafting a Pitch," *Kelly J. Baker: Cold Takes*, https://perma.cc/G65X-CDHB, accessed April 1, 2023, http://www.kellyjbaker.com/crafting-a-pitch/.

CHAPTER 8. WRITING DEPRESSION

1. William Styron, *Darkness Visible: A Memoir of Madness* (New York: Random House, 1990), 82.

2. Giulia Perini et al., "Cognitive Impairment in Depression: Recent Advances and Novel Treatments," *Neuropsychiatric Disease and Treatment* 15 (May 2019): 1250, https://doi.org/10.2147/NDT.S199746.

3. Katie Rose Guest Pryal, "Depression, The Essay," March 19, 2019, *Katie Rose Guest Pryal*, https://katieroseguestpryal.com/2019/03/19/depression-the-essay/.

4. Stella Young, "I'm Not Your Inspiration, Thank You Very Much," *TEDxSydney*, June 9, 2014, https://perma.cc/W6P3-ZZVX, https://www.ted.com/talks/stella_young_i_m_not_your_inspiration_thank_you_very_much.

5. *A Beautiful Mind*, directed by Ron Howard (Universal City, CA: Universal Pictures, 2001).

6. *Captain America: Civil War*, directed by Anthony and Joe Russo (Burbank, CA: Marvel Studios, 2016).

7. Katie Rose Guest Pryal, "My Disability Story Isn't for Your Catharsis," *The Establishment*, September 25, 2018, https://perma.cc/V7Z8-6UGR, https://theestablishment.co/my-disability-story-isnt-for-your-catharsis/index.html.

CHAPTER 9. "THE DARKNESS THAT IS PLAGUING OUR UNIVERSITY"

1. Kevin M. Guskiewicz, "FORMAL NOTICE: World Mental Health Day; Classes Canceled Oct 12," Email, October 10, 2021.

2. Part of the reason colleges seemed eager to ignore the crisis, especially in 2021, was their desire to get students back to campus after the COVID shutdown. College administrations rushed to reopen on-campus instruction for financial reasons. This rush included a push to fill residence halls, which lost money every day they sat empty. Colleges suffered massive financial losses due to COVID. One research study estimated "$85 billion in lost revenues, $24 billion for Covid-related expenses, and $74 billion in anticipated future decreases in state funding. That adds up to a whopping $183 billion." Paul M. Friga, "How Much Has Covid Cost Colleges? $183 Billion," *Chronicle of Higher Education*, February 5, 2021, https://perma.cc/6T3B-9596, https://www.chronicle.com/article/how-to-fight-covids-financial-crush.

3. Qijin Cheng et al., "Suicide Contagion: A Systematic Review of Definitions and Research Utility," ed. Martin Voracek, *PLoS ONE* 9, no. 9 (September 26, 2014): e108724.

4. Ben Kesslen, "UNC Chapel Hill Cancels Classes Tuesday amid Two Suicide Investigations," *NBC News*, October 11, 2021, https://perma.cc/WH38-Z434, https://www.nbcnews.com/news/us-news/unc-chapel-hill-cancels-classes-tuesday-amid-two-suicide-investigations-n1281229.

5. Kesslen, "UNC Chapel Hill Cancels Classes."

6. Alex Findijs, "UNC Chapel Hill Campus Mourns Suicide and Attempted Suicide of Two Students over the Weekend," *World Socialist Web Site*, October 14, 2021, https://perma.cc/R7L4-QJDJ, https://www.wsws.org/en/articles/2021/10/15/unca-o15.html.

7. UNC Police, "Crime Log," *University of North Carolina at Chapel Hill*, https://perma.cc/6V8Y-HN4L, accessed March 23, 2023, https://p2c.police.unc.edu/crime-log/.

8. Law Dictionary, "What Is a Police Welfare Check?" *The Law Dictionary*, accessed April 1, 2023, https://thelawdictionary.org/article/what-is-a-police-welfare-check/.

9. Healthy Minds Network, "Fall 2020 Data Report," *Healthy Minds Study*, Fall 2020, 10, https://perma.cc/9XWA-2DF8, https://healthymindsnetwork.org/wp-content/uploads/2021/02/HMS-Fall-2020-National-Data-Report.pdf.

10. Julius Miller, "Stanford Responds to Suicide Crisis after 4th Student in 13 Months Takes Her Own Life," *Los Angeles Magazine*, March 11, 2022, https://perma.cc/83A7-CZ5E, https://www.lamag.com/article/stanford-responds-to-suicide-crisis-after-4th-student-in-13-months-takes-her-own-life/.

11. Chelsea Donovan and Aaron Thomas, "Two NC State Students Died by Suicide within 24 Hours; Counseling Services to Be Offered Friday,"

WRAL.Com, https://perma.cc/W4H4-SFDS, accessed April 28, 2023, https://legacy.wral.com/two-nc-state-students-died-by-suicide-within-24-hours-counseling-services-to-be-offered-friday/20831899/.

12. Danielle R. Busby et al., "Black College Students at Elevated Risk for Suicide: Barriers to Mental Health Service Utilization," *Journal of American College Health* 69, no. 3 (April 3, 2021): 311.

13. Busby et al., 311.

14. Busby et al., 312.

15. Busby et al., 313.

16. Busby et al., 313.

17. Asian American Psychological Association Leadership Fellows Program, "Suicide among Asian Americans," *American Psychological Association*, May 2012, https://www.apa.org/pi/oema/resources/ethnicity-health/asian-american/suicide-fact-sheet.pdf.

18. Jenn Fang, "Asian American Student Suicide Rate at MIT Is Quadruple the National Average," *Reappropriate: Asian American Feminism, Politics, and Pop Culture*, May 20, 2015, https://perma.cc/NK6X-V6QU, http://reappropriate.co/2015/05/asian-american-student-suicide-rate-at-mit-is-quadruple-the-national-average/.

19. Uwill, "About Us," *Uwill: Student Mental Health & Wellness*, accessed April 1, 2023, https://uwill.com/about-us/.

20. Maria Carrasco, "Colleges Seek Virtual Mental Health Services," *Inside Higher Ed*, September 20, 2021, https://perma.cc/P3UD-EVH9, https://www.insidehighered.com/news/2021/09/20/colleges-expand-mental-health-services-students.

21. Katie Rose Guest Pryal, "Front-Line Faculty and Systemic Burnout: Why More Faculty Should Attend to Law Students' Mental Health and the Inequities Caused by Faculty Who Opt Out," *Legal Writing: The Journal of the Legal Writing Institute* 27, no. 1 (2023): 199–221.

22. Eric Westervelt, "Mental Health and Police Violence: How Crisis Intervention Teams Are Failing," *NPR*, September 18, 2020, https://perma.cc/U7CM-8ZU2, https://www.npr.org/2020/09/18/913229469/mental-health-and-police-violence-how-crisis-intervention-teams-are-failing.

23. Emilie Poplett, "Carolina Launches 24/7 Hotline to Support Student Mental Health," *The University of North Carolina at Chapel Hill*, August 19, 2019, https://perma.cc/AX54-KQ7V, https://www.unc.edu/posts/2019/08/19/carolina-launches-24-7-hotline-to-support-student-mental-health/.

24. Healthy Minds Network, "Fall 2020 Data Report," 10.

25. Katie J. M. Baker, "How Colleges Flunk Mental Health," *Newsweek*, February 11, 2014, https://perma.cc/V4JD-47ML, https://www.newsweek.com/2014/02/14/how-colleges-flunk-mental-health-245492.html.

26. Baker, "How Colleges Flunk Mental Health."

27. Esmé Weijun Wang, *The Collected Schizophrenias* (Minneapolis, MN: Graywolf Press, 2019), 73.

28. Abigail Napp and Harsha Nahata, "When Colleges Fail on Mental Health," *NYCITY NewsService of the CUNY Craig Newmark Graduate School of Journalism*, May 5, 2020, https://perma.cc/N45N-MBTA, https://campus mentalhealth.nycitynewsservice.com/.

29. Elizabeth Pham Janowski, "Sent Away," *Chronicle of Higher Education*, June 27, 2022, https://www.chronicle.com/article/sent-away.

30. Janowski, "Sent Away."

31. Ilanit Tal Young et al., "Suicide Bereavement and Complicated Grief," *Dialogues in Clinical Neuroscience* 14, no. 2 (June 30, 2012): 180, https://doi .org/10.31887/DCNS.2012.14.2/iyoung.

32. Robert E. Litman, "Medical-Legal Aspects of Suicide," *Washburn Law Journal* 6, no. 2 (Winter 1967): 395. The nine states were Alabama, Kentucky, New Jersey, North Carolina, North Dakota, Oklahoma, South Carolina, South Dakota, and Washington.

33. University of North Carolina Graduate and Professional Student Government Executive Board and University of North Carolina Undergraduate Student Government Executive Board, "Call for a Pause to Instruction," Letter, October 10, 2021.

34. Lamar Richards, "Lamar Richards, Tweet as UNC Student Body President, Stating Students Need a Break from Classes the Day after the Announcement of Multiple Student Deaths by Suicide," Twitter, October 10, 2021.

35. Chronicle of Higher Education Editors, "How to Solve the Student-Disengagement Crisis," *Chronicle of Higher Education*, May 11, 2022, https:// perma.cc/E98H-B7UN, https://www.chronicle.com/article/how-to-solve-the -student-disengagement-crisis.

CHAPTER 10. RIGOR ANGST

1. Dan Berrett, "The Making of a Teaching Evangelist," *Chronicle of Higher Education*, June 5, 2016, https://www.chronicle.com/article/the-making-of-a -teaching-evangelist/.

2. Aleszu Bajak, "Lectures Aren't Just Boring, They're Ineffective, Too, Study Finds," *Science*, May 12, 2014, https://perma.cc/3V7J-8BVQ, https://www .science.org/content/article/lectures-arent-just-boring-theyre-ineffective-too -study-finds. Bajak's article refers to the following study: Scott Freeman et al., "Active Learning Increases Student Performance in Science, Engineering, and Mathematics," *Proceedings of the National Academy of Sciences of the United States of America* 111, no. 23 (June 2014): 8410–8415, https://doi.org/10.1073 /pnas.1319030111.

3. Berrett, "The Making of a Teaching Evangelist."

4. Beckie Supiano, "A Different Way of Thinking about Rigor," *Chronicle of Higher Education*, November 18, 2021, https://www.chronicle.com/newsletter/teaching/2021-11-18.

5. Jordynn Jack and Viji Sathy, "It's Time to Cancel the Word 'Rigor,'" *Chronicle of Higher Education*, September 24, 2021, https://perma.cc/ERV2-5DAW, https://www.chronicle.com/article/its-time-to-cancel-the-word-rigor.

6. Jack and Sathy, "It's Time to Cancel the Word 'Rigor.'"

7. H. Holden Thorp, "Inclusion Doesn't Lower Standards," *Science* 377, no. 6602 (July 8, 2022): 129.

8. Deborah J. Cohan, "Upholding Rigor at Pandemic U," *Inside Higher Ed*, August 25, 2021, https://perma.cc/NMP8-XZCE, https://www.insidehighered.com/advice/2021/08/25/professors-should-uphold-rigor-when-assessing-students-even-pandemic-opinion.

9. Aja Romano, "A History of 'Wokeness,'" *Vox*, October 9, 2020, https://perma.cc/33TM-4SEH, https://www.vox.com/culture/21437879/stay-woke-wokeness-history-origin-evolution-controversy.

10. Cohan, "Upholding Rigor at Pandemic U."

11. Cohan, "Upholding Rigor at Pandemic U."

12. Cohan, "Upholding Rigor at Pandemic U."

13. David Randall, "Don't Cancel Rigor," *National Association of Scholars*, November 4, 2021, https://perma.cc/7DL2-Z42Q, https://www.nas.org/blogs/article/dont-cancel-rigor.

14. Beckie Supiano, "The Redefinition of Rigor," *Chronicle of Higher Education*, March 29, 2022, https://perma.cc/2XGW-WTJS, https://www.chronicle.com/article/the-redefinition-of-rigor.

15. Kevin Gannon, reported by Supiano, "The Redefinition of Rigor." Gannon expands on his ideas in Kevin Gannon, "Why Calls for a 'Return to Rigor' Are Wrong," *Chronicle of Higher Education*, May 22, 2023, https://www.chronicle.com/article/why-calls-for-a-return-to-rigor-are-wrong.

16. Supiano, "The Redefinition of Rigor."

17. Kevin Gannon, "Post-Covid, the Personal Is the Professional," *Chronicle of Higher Education*, April 4, 2022, https://www.chronicle.com/article/post-covid-the-personal-is-the-professional.

18. Brooks and McGurk, reported by Supiano, "The Redefinition of Rigor."

19. Mays Imad, "Hope Matters," *Inside Higher Ed*, March 17, 2020, https://perma.cc/FH89-LYED, https://www.insidehighered.com/advice/2020/03/17/10-strategies-support-students-and-help-them-learn-during-coronavirus-crisis.

20. Karen Ray Costa, "Tweet Coining the Term 'Toxic Rigor,'" Twitter, December 9, 2020. See also a discussion of the topic in Karen Ray Costa, "The Next Phase," *Karen Ray Costa*, May 19, 2021, https://karenraycosta.medium.com/the-next-phase-a7912bc6a453.

21. Lee Skallerup Bessette, "Can You Teach a 'Transformative' Humanities Course Online?" *Chronicle of Higher Education*, July 9, 2020, https://perma.cc/BMM3-U3UF, https://www.chronicle.com/article/can-you-teach-a-transformative-humanities-course-online.

22. Bessette, "Can You Teach a 'Transformative' Humanities Course Online?"

23. Bryan M. Dewsbury et al., "Inclusive and Active Pedagogies Reduce Academic Outcome Gaps and Improve Long-Term Performance," *PLOS ONE* 17, no. 6 (June 15, 2022): e0268620.

24. Tweet by Bryan M. Dewsbury quoted in Beckie Supiano, "Worried about Cutting Content? This Study Suggests It's OK," *Chronicle of Higher Education*, July 7, 2022, https://www.chronicle.com/newsletter/teaching/2022-07-07.

CHAPTER 11. TOXIC RIGOR IS ABLEIST

1. Beckie Supiano, "The Redefinition of Rigor," *Chronicle of Higher Education*, March 29, 2022, https://perma.cc/2XGW-WTJS, https://www.chronicle.com/article/the-redefinition-of-rigor.

2. Karen Ray Costa, "Tweet Coining the Term 'Toxic Rigor,'" Twitter, December 9, 2020. See also a discussion of the topic in Karen Ray Costa, "The Next Phase," *Karen Ray Costa*, May 19, 2021, https://karenraycosta.medium.com/the-next-phase-a7912bc6a453.

3. David Randall, "Don't Cancel Rigor," *National Association of Scholars*, November 4, 2021, https://perma.cc/7DL2-Z42Q, https://www.nas.org/blogs/article/dont-cancel-rigor.

4. Randall is responding to Jordynn Jack and Viji Sathy, "It's Time to Cancel the Word 'Rigor,'" *Chronicle of Higher Education*, September 24, 2021, https://perma.cc/ERV2-5DAW, https://www.chronicle.com/article/its-time-to-cancel-the-word-rigor.

5. Pradeep K. Dubey and John Geanakoplos, "Grading Exams: 100, 99, 98, . . . Or A, B, C?," *SSRN Scholarly Paper* (Rochester, NY, June 18, 2009).

6. Jonathan Malesic, "My College Students Are Not OK," *New York Times*, May 13, 2022, https://perma.cc/V65W-PXXS, https://www.nytimes.com/2022/05/13/opinion/college-university-remote-pandemic.html.

7. Deborah J. Cohan, "Upholding Rigor at Pandemic U," *Inside Higher Ed*, August 25, 2021, https://perma.cc/NMP8-XZCE, https://www.insidehighered.com/advice/2021/08/25/professors-should-uphold-rigor-when-assessing-students-even-pandemic-opinion.

8. Doron Dorfman, "Fear of the Disability Con: Perceptions of Fraud and Special Rights Discourse," *Law and Society Review* 53, no. 4 (December 2019): 1053.

9. Dorfman, "Fear of the Disability Con," 1051.

10. Katherine A. Macfarlane, "Accommodation Discrimination," *American University Law Review*, 72 (forthcoming 2023), 27.

11. Macfarlane, "Accommodation Discrimination," 19.

12. Dorfman, "Fear of the Disability Con," 1061.

13. Katie Rose Guest Pryal and Jordynn Jack, "When You Talk about Banning Laptops, You Throw Disabled Students Under the Bus," *The Huffington Post*, November 27, 2017.

14. Dorfman, "Fear of the Disability Con," 1078.

15. Dorfman, "Fear of the Disability Con," 1079.

16. Jay Timothy Dolmage, *Academic Ableism: Disability and Higher Education* (Ann Arbor: University of Michigan Press, 2017), 10.

17. Margaret Price, *Mad at School, Rhetorics of Mental Disability and Academic Life* (Ann Arbor: University of Michigan Press, 2011), 130.

18. Ayla Samli and Katie Rose Guest Pryal, "Accommodations Are Not Accessibility: An Interview with Katie Rose Guest Pryal," *The Rumpus*, September 21, 2022, https://perma.cc/JR6G-5VTM, https://therumpus.net/2022/09/21/accommodations-are-not-accessibility-an-interview-with-katie-rose-guest-pryal/.

19. Gail A. Hornstein, "Why I Dread the Accommodations Talk," *Chronicle of Higher Education*, March 26, 2017, https://perma.cc/PP73-8WKJ, https://www.chronicle.com/article/Why-I-Dread-the-Accommodations/239571.

20. Hornstein, "Why I Dread the Accommodations Talk."

21. Hornstein, "Why I Dread the Accommodations Talk."

22. Adam Grant, "Why We Should Stop Grading Students on a Curve," *New York Times*, September 10, 2016, https://perma.cc/Z6SS-C5DF, https://www.nytimes.com/2016/09/11/opinion/sunday/why-we-should-stop-grading-students-on-a-curve.html.

23. Kaci Bishop, "Framing Failure in the Legal Classroom: Techniques for Encouraging Growth and Resilience," *Arkansas Law Review* 70, no. 4 (2018): 959–1005.

24. Sarah J. Schendel, "Due Dates in the Real World: Extensions, Equity, and the Hidden Curriculum," *The Georgetown Journal of Legal Ethics* 35, no. 2 (2022): 205.

CHAPTER 12. TEACHING MENTALLY DISABLED STUDENTS

1. Cornell University, "Universal Design for Learning," *Cornell Center for Teaching Innovation*, accessed March 26, 2023, https://teaching.cornell.edu/teaching-resources/designing-your-course/universal-design-learning.

2. Susan W. White, Thomas H. Ollendick, and Bethany C. Bray, "College Students on the Autism Spectrum: Prevalence and Associated Problems," *Autism* 15, no. 6 (November 1, 2011): 683–701.

3. Arthur D. P. Mak et al., "ADHD Comorbidity Structure and Impairment: Results of the WHO World Mental Health Surveys International College

Student Project (WMH-ICS)," *Journal of Attention Disorders* 26, no. 8 (June 1, 2022): 1078–1096.

4. Kasey Meeks, Amy Sutton Peak, and Adam Dreihaus, "Depression, Anxiety, and Stress among Students, Faculty, and Staff," *Journal of American College Health* 71, no. 2 (February 12, 2023): 348–354.

5. ADDitude Editors, "Your Executive Functions Are Weak; Here's Why," *ADDitude Magazine*, April 13, 2022, https://www.additudemag.com/slideshows/what-are-adhd-executive-functions/.

6. Maggie Coughlin, "10 Things Faculty Need to Understand about Autism," *Inside Higher Ed*, October 20, 2021, https://www.insidehighered.com/advice/2021/10/20/lessons-teaching-students-autism-spectrum-opinion.

7. Jennifer C. Sarrett, "Autism and Accommodations in Higher Education: Insights from the Autism Community," *Journal of Autism and Developmental Disorders* 48, no. 3 (March 2018): 681.

8. Kathleen E. Hupfeld, Tessa R. Abagis, and Priti Shah, "Living 'in the Zone': Hyperfocus in Adult ADHD," *ADHD Attention Deficit and Hyperactivity Disorders* 11, no. 2 (June 1, 2019): 191–208.

9. Doron Dorfman, "Fear of the Disability Con: Perceptions of Fraud and Special Rights Discourse," *Law and Society Review* 53, no. 4 (December 2019): 1051–1091.

10. ADDitude Editors, "What NOT to Say to the Parent of a Child with ADHD," *ADDitude Magazine*, September 28, 2021, https://perma.cc/E7RK-4JZL, https://www.additudemag.com/slideshows/common-myths-about-adhd/.

11. Katherine Macfarlane, "Accommodation Discrimination (Preprint)," *American University Law Review* 72 (2023).

12. Christopher Toutain, "Barriers to Accommodations for Students with Disabilities in Higher Education: A Literature Review," *Journal of Postsecondary Education and Disability* 32, no. 3 (Fall 2019): 300.

13. Robert McCrossin, "Finding the True Number of Females with Autistic Spectrum Disorder by Estimating the Biases in Initial Recognition and Clinical Diagnosis," *Children (Basel, Switzerland)* 9, no. 2 (February 17, 2022), 272.

14. White, Ollendick, and Bray, "College Students on the Autism Spectrum."

15. Stephanie Pinder-Amaker, "Identifying the Unmet Needs of College Students on the Autism Spectrum," *Harvard Review of Psychiatry* 22, no. 2 (2014): 125–137.

16. Eric Garcia, *We're Not Broken: Changing the Autism Conversation* (Boston: Houghton Mifflin Harcourt, 2021), 35.

17. Kimberly S. Austin and Edlyn Vallejo Peña, "Exceptional Faculty Members Who Responsively Teach Students with Autism Spectrum Disorders," *Journal of Postsecondary Education and Disability* 30, no. 1 (2017): 26.

18. Keith Low, "What Is Executive Function?" *Verywell Mind*, September 27, 2020, https://www.verywellmind.com/what-are-executive-functions-20463.

19. Kelly A. Hogan and Viji Sathy, *Inclusive Teaching: Strategies for*

Promoting Equity in the College Classroom (Morgantown: West Virginia University Press, 2022), 43.

20. Randall W. Engle, "What Is Working Memory Capacity?" in *The Nature of Remembering: Essays in Honor of Robert G. Crowder*, ed. Henry L. Roediger, et al. (Washington, DC: American Psychological Association, 2001), 297–314.

21. Hogan and Sathy, *Inclusive Teaching*, 44.

22. Hogan and Sathy, *Inclusive Teaching*, 44.

23. Stimpunks, "Eye Contact and Neurodiversity," *Stimpunks Foundation*, March 2, 2023, https://stimpunks.org/eye-contact/.

24. Stimpunks, "Eye Contact and Neurodiversity."

25. Fiona G. Phelps, Gwyneth Doherty-Sneddon, and Hannah Warnock, "Helping Children Think: Gaze Aversion and Teaching," *British Journal of Developmental Psychology* 24, no. 3 (2006): 577–588.

26. Joan M. McGuire and Sally S. Scott, "An Approach for Inclusive College Teaching: Universal Design for Instruction," *Learning Disabilities: A Multidisciplinary Journal* 14, no. 1 (2006): 21–32.

27. McGuire and Scott, "An Approach for Inclusive College Teaching," 27.

28. Low, "What Is Executive Function?"

29. Garcia, *We're Not Broken*, 36.

30. Coughlin, "10 Things Faculty Need to Understand About Autism."

CHAPTER 13. FRONT-LINE FACULTY

1. Katie Rose Guest Pryal, "Front-Line Faculty and Systemic Burnout: Why More Faculty Should Attend to Law Students' Mental Health and the Inequities Caused by Faculty Who Opt Out," *Legal Writing: The Journal of the Legal Writing Institute* 27, no. 1 (2023): 199–221.

2. Katie Rose Guest Pryal, *Life of the Mind Interrupted: Essays on Mental Health and Disability in Higher Education* (Chapel Hill, NC: Blue Crow Books, 2017), 141.

3. For more, see Victoria McDermott et al., eds., *On the Front Lines: Women Educators' Experiences during the COVID-19 Pandemic* (Lanham, MD: Lexington Books, 2023).

4. "For example, one study found that although both male and female undergraduate associate professors averaged a sixty-four-hour work week, institutional service work and other institutional commitments resulted in the women professors having 220 fewer hours than their male counterparts to devote to scholarly endeavors during the academic year." Andrea A. Curcio and Mary A. Lynch, "Addressing Social Loafing on Faculty Committees," *Journal of Legal Education* 67, no. 1 (Autumn 2017): 249.

5. Meera E. Deo, "Pandemic Pressures on Faculty," *University of Pennsylvania Law Review Online* 170, no. 1 (2022): 130.

6. Deo, "Pandemic Pressures on Faculty," 130.

7. Alexa Z. Chew and Rachel Gurvich, "Saying the Quiet Parts Out Loud: Teaching Students How Law School Works," *Nebraska Law Review* 100, no. 4 (2021): 887–904.

8. Margaret Price, *Mad at School, Rhetorics of Mental Disability and Academic Life* (Ann Arbor: University of Michigan Press, 2011), 26.

9. Katie Rose Guest Pryal, "Disclosure Blues: Should You Tell Colleagues about Your Mental Illness?" *Chronicle of Higher Education*, June 13, 2014.

10. Sarah J. Schendel, "The Pandemic Syllabus," *Denver Law Review Forum*, November 30, 2020, https://perma.cc/2FUH-DNUJ, https://www.denverlaw review.org/dlr-online-article/pandemicsyllabus.

11. Interview with Teresa Heinz Housel via video conference, March 8, 2023.

CHAPTER 14. PROCRASTINATION AND COMPASSION

1. Sarah J. Schendel, "Due Dates in the Real World: Extensions, Equity, and the Hidden Curriculum," *The Georgetown Journal of Legal Ethics* 35, no. 2 (2022): 205.

2. Alison L. Flett, Mohsen Haghbin, and Timothy A. Pychyl, "Procrastination and Depression from a Cognitive Perspective: An Exploration of the Associations among Procrastinatory Automatic Thoughts, Rumination, and Mindfulness," *The Journal of Rational-Emotive and Cognitive-Behavior Therapy* 34, no. 3 (September 2016): 170.

3. Devon Price, "Laziness Does Not Exist," *Human Parts*, March 23, 2018, https://perma.cc/LZ8J-LXWU, https://humanparts.medium.com/laziness-does -not-exist-3af27e312do1. See also, Devon Price, *Laziness Does Not Exist: A Defense of the Exhausted, Exploited, and Overworked* (New York: Simon and Schuster, 2021).

4. Flett, Haghbin, and Pychyl, "Procrastination and Depression," 180.

5. Flett, Haghbin, and Pychyl, "Procrastination and Depression," 171.

6. Flett, Haghbin, and Pychyl, "Procrastination and Depression," 182.

7. Flett, Haghbin, and Pychyl, "Procrastination and Depression," 181.

8. Flett, Haghbin, and Pychyl, "Procrastination and Depression," 182.

9. Flett, Haghbin, and Pychyl, "Procrastination and Depression," 173.

10. Kristin Neff, "Self-Compassion: An Alternative Conceptualization of a Healthy Attitude toward Oneself," *Self and Identity* 2, no. 2 (2003): 87.

11. Neff, "Self-Compassion," 87

12. Kristin D. Neff, Ya-Ping Hsieh, and Kullaya Dejitterat, "Self-Compassion, Achievement Goals, and Coping with Academic Failure," *Self and Identity* 4, no. 3 (July 2005): 263–287.

13. Neff, Hsieh, and Dejitterat, "Self-Compassion, Achievement Goals, and Coping with Academic Failure," 272.

14. Neff, Hsieh, and Dejitterat, "Self-Compassion, Achievement Goals, and Coping with Academic Failure," 284.

15. Neff, Hsieh, and Dejitterat, "Self-Compassion, Achievement Goals, and Coping with Academic Failure," 89.

16. Schendel, "Due Dates in the Real World," 226–227.

17. Schendel, "Due Dates in the Real World," 227.

18. Kaci Bishop, "Framing Failure in the Legal Classroom: Techniques for Encouraging Growth and Resilience," *Arkansas Law Review* 70, no. 4 (2018): 969.

19. Bishop, "Framing Failure in the Legal Classroom," 970.

20. Bishop, "Framing Failure in the Legal Classroom," 970.

CHAPTER 15. TEACHING ACCESSIBLY/INCLUSIVELY

1. I am referring to "toxic rigor," a term coined by Karen Ray Costa. Costa, "Tweet Coining the Term 'Toxic Rigor,'" Twitter, December 9, 2020. See also a discussion of the topic in Karen Ray Costa, "The Next Phase," *Karen Ray Costa*, May 19, 2021, https://karenraycosta.medium.com/the-next-phase -a7912bc6a453.

2. Jay Timothy Dolmage, *Academic Ableism: Disability in Higher Education* (Ann Arbor: University of Michigan Press, 2017): 118–119. Dolmage gives credit to Star Ford, "Deep Accessibility," *Ianology*, September 6, 2013, https://perma .cc/AN42-J8TM, https://ianology.wordpress.com/2013/09/06/deep-accessibil ity/.

3. Catherine J. Denial, "A Pedagogy of Kindness," *Hybrid Pedagogy*, August 15, 2019, https://hybridpedagogy.org/pedagogy-of-kindness/.

4. Beckie Supiano, "The Redefinition of Rigor," *Chronicle of Higher Education*, March 29, 2022, https://perma.cc/2XGW-WTJS, https://www.chronicle .com/article/the-redefinition-of-rigor.

5. Jonathan Malesic, "My College Students Are Not OK," *New York Times*, May 13, 2022, https://perma.cc/V65W-PXXS, https://www.nytimes .com/2022/05/13/opinion/college-university-remote-pandemic.html.

6. Matthew Cortland, "Why Banning Laptops Is Harmful," *Education in Chemistry*, October 6, 2017, https://perma.cc/9783-J6F3, https://edu.rsc.org /endpoint/why-banning-laptops-is-harmful/3008076.article.

7. Pam A. Mueller and Daniel M. Oppenheimer, "The Pen Is Mightier than the Keyboard: Advantages of Longhand over Laptop Note Taking," *Psychological Science* 25, no. 6 (June 1, 2014): 1159–1168, https://doi .org/10.1177/0956797614524581.

8. Heather L. Urry et al., "Don't Ditch the Laptop Just Yet: A Direct Replication of Mueller and Oppenheimer's (2014) Study 1 Plus Mini Meta-Analyses across Similar Studies," *Psychological Science* 32, no. 3 (March 1, 2021): 326–339, https://doi.org/10.1177/0956797620965541.

9. Urry et al., "Don't Ditch the Laptop Just Yet," 326.

10. Katie Rose Guest Pryal and Jordynn Jack, "When You Talk about Banning Laptops, You Throw Disabled Students under the Bus," *Huffington Post*, November 27, 2017, https://ssrn.com/abstract=4166867 or http://dx.doi.org /10.2139/ssrn.4166867.

11. Denial, "A Pedagogy of Kindness."

12. Cortland, "Why Banning Laptops Is Harmful."

13. Cortland, "Why Banning Laptops Is Harmful."

14. Pryal and Jack, "When You Talk about Banning Laptops."

15. Ellen Boucher, "It's Time to Ditch Our Deadlines," *The Chronicle of Higher Education*, August 22, 2016, https://www.chronicle.com/article/its-time-to -ditch-our-deadlines/.

16. Sarah J. Schendel, "Due Dates in the Real World: Extensions, Equity, and the Hidden Curriculum," *Georgetown Journal of Legal Ethics* 35, no. 2 (2022): 205.

17. Schendel, "Due Dates in the Real World," 226.

18. Schendel, "Due Dates in the Real World," 226.

19. Interview with Teresa Heinz Housel via video conference, March 8, 2023.

20. Eric Garcia, *We're Not Broken: Changing the Autism Conversation* (Boston: Houghton Mifflin Harcourt, 2021), 39.

21. Garcia, *We're Not Broken*, 39.

22. Denial, "A Pedagogy of Kindness."

23. Interview in person, September 2022.

24. Denial, "A Pedagogy of Kindness."

25. Michael Bérubé, "Cut Students Some Slack Already," *Chronicle of Higher Education*, May 4, 2022, https://www.chronicle.com/article/cut-students -some-slack-already.

26. Vini Olsen-Reeder, "Commentary: 'Plumbing Leaks: The Post-Pandemic Neoliberal Turn of Tertiary Students,'" *New Zealand Journal of Educational Studies*, December 15, 2022.

27. Interview by email, March 28, 2023.

28. Doron Dorfman, "Fear of the Disability Con: Perceptions of Fraud and Special Rights Discourse," *Law and Society Review* 53, no. 4 (December 2019): 1053.

29. Katherine A. Macfarlane, "Accommodation Discrimination," *American University Law Review*, 72 (forthcoming 2023), 27.

Bibliography

ADDitude Editors. "What NOT to Say to the Parent of a Child with ADHD." *ADDitude Magazine*, September 28, 2021. https://perma.cc/E7RK-4JZL. https://www.additudemag.com/slideshows/common-myths-about-adhd/.

ADDitude Editors. "Your Executive Functions Are Weak. Here's Why." *ADDitude Magazine*, April 13, 2022. https://www.additudemag.com/slideshows/what-are-adhd-executive-functions/.

Allen, Renee Nicole, Alicia Jackson, and DeShun Harris. "The 'Pink Ghetto' Pipeline: Challenges and Opportunities for Women in Legal Education." *University of Detroit Mercy Law Review* 96, no. 2 (Summer 2019): 525–555.

American Psychiatric Association. "What Is Mental Illness?" *American Psychiatric Association*. https://perma.cc/B47X-3K6N. Accessed March 24, 2023. https://psychiatry.org/patients-families/what-is-mental-illness.

Asian American Psychological Association Leadership Fellows Program. "Suicide among Asian Americans." *American Psychological Association*, May 2012. https://www.apa.org/pi/oema/resources/ethnicity-health/asian-american/suicide-fact-sheet.pdf.

Austin, Kimberly S., and Edlyn Vallejo Peña. "Exceptional Faculty Members Who Responsively Teach Students with Autism Spectrum Disorders." *Journal of Postsecondary Education and Disability* 30, no. 1 (2017): 17–32.

Bajak, Aleszu. "Lectures Aren't Just Boring, They're Ineffective, Too, Study Finds." *Science*, May 12, 2014. https://perma.cc/3V7J-8BVQ. https://www.science.org/content/article/lectures-arent-just-boring-theyre-ineffective-too-study-finds.

Baker, Katie J. M. "How Colleges Flunk Mental Health." *Newsweek*, February 11, 2014. https://perma.cc/V4JD-47ML. https://www.newsweek.com/2014/02/14/how-colleges-flunk-mental-health-245492.html.

Baker, Kelly J. "Crafting a Pitch." *Kelly J. Baker: Cold Takes*. https://perma.cc/G65X-CDHB. Accessed April 1, 2023. http://www.kellyjbaker.com/crafting-a-pitch/.

———. *Sexism Ed: Essays on Gender and Labor in Academia*. Chapel Hill, NC: Blue Crow Books, 2018.

Belcher, Hannah. "Autistic People and Masking." *National Autistic Society (UK)*, July 7, 2022. https://perma.cc/68PT-E2N2. https://www.autism.org .uk/advice-and-guidance/professional-practice/autistic-masking.

Bergen, Clara, Lisa Bortolotti, Katherine Tallent, Matthew Broome, Michael Larkin, Rachel Temple, Catherine Fadashe, Carmen Lee, Michele C. Lim, and Rose McCabe. "Communication in Youth Mental Health Clinical Encounters: Introducing the Agential Stance." *Theory and Psychology* 32, no. 5 (October 2022): 667–690. https://doi.org/10.1177/09593543221095079.

Berrett, Dan. "The Making of a Teaching Evangelist." *Chronicle of Higher Education*, June 5, 2016. https://www.chronicle.com/article/the-making-of-a -teaching-evangelist/.

Bérubé, Michael. "Cut Students Some Slack Already." *Chronicle of Higher Education*, May 4, 2022. https://www.chronicle.com/article/cut-students-some -slack-already.

Bessette, Lee Skallerup. "Can You Teach a 'Transformative' Humanities Course Online?" *Chronicle of Higher Education*, July 9, 2020. https://perma.cc /BMM3-U3UF.https://www.chronicle.com/article/can-you-teach-a-transform ative-humanities-course-online.

Bishop, Kaci. "Framing Failure in the Legal Classroom: Techniques for Encouraging Growth and Resilience." *Arkansas Law Review* 70, no. 4 (2018): 959–1005.

Boucher, Ellen. "It's Time to Ditch Our Deadlines." *Chronicle of Higher Education*, August 22, 2016. https://www.chronicle.com/article/its-time-to-ditch -our-deadlines/.

Bousquet, Marc. "The Rhetoric of 'Job Market' and the Reality of the Academic Labor System." *College English* 66, no. 2 (November 2003): 207–228. https:// doi.org/10.2307/3594266.

Brown, Lydia X. Z. "Ableism/Language." *Autistic Hoya*, September 14, 2022. http://autistichoya.com/ableist-words-and-terms-to-avoid.html.

——. "Identity-First Language." *Autistic Self Advocacy Network*, March 2, 2012. https://perma.cc/5L6C-7SDM. https://autisticadvocacy.org/about -asan/identity-first-language/.

Busby, Danielle R., Kai Zheng, Daniel Eisenberg, Ronald C. Albucher, Todd Favorite, William Coryell, Jacqueline Pistorello, and Cheryl A. King. "Black College Students at Elevated Risk for Suicide: Barriers to Mental Health Service Utilization." *Journal of American College Health* 69, no. 3 (April 3, 2021): 308–314. https://doi.org/10.1080/07448481.2019.1674316.

Carrasco, Maria. "Colleges Seek Virtual Mental Health Services." *Inside Higher Ed*, September 20, 2021. https://perma.cc/P3UD-EVH9. https://www.in sidehighered.com/news/2021/09/20/colleges-expand-mental-health -services-students.

Centers for Disease Control and Prevention. "Facts about Developmental

Disabilities." *CDC*. https://perma.cc/5MK4-TWKC. Accessed March 23, 2023. https://www.cdc.gov/ncbddd/developmentaldisabilities/facts.html.

———. "What Is Autism Spectrum Disorder?" *CDC*. https://perma.cc/PKV6 -2U7H. Accessed March 23, 2023. https://www.cdc.gov/ncbddd/autism /facts.html.

Chang, Anna. "MLA Publishes New Guidelines on Evaluating Publicly Engaged Humanities Scholarship." *MLA Commons*, August 17, 2022. https://perma .cc/PPP9-87B3. https://news.mla.hcommons.org/2022/08/17/mla-publish es-new-guidelines-on-evaluating-publicly-engaged-humanities-scholar ship/.

Cheng, Qijin, Hong Li, Vincent Silenzio, and Eric D. Caine. "Suicide Contagion: A Systematic Review of Definitions and Research Utility." Edited by Mar- tin Voracek. *PLoS ONE* 9, no. 9 (September 26, 2014): e108724. https://doi .org/10.1371/journal.pone.0108724.

Cherry, Kendra. "What Is the Illusion of Control?" *Verywell Mind*, August 3, 2022. https://perma.cc/K39T-M2CC. https://www.verywellmind.com/what -is-the-illusion-of-control-5198406.

Chew, Alexa Z., and Rachel Gurvich. "Saying the Quiet Parts Out Loud: Teach- ing Students How Law School Works." Nebraska Law Review 100, no. 4 (2021): 887–904.

Choi, Kristen R., MarySue V. Heilemann, Alex Fauer, and Meredith Mead. "A Second Pandemic: Mental Health Spillover from the Novel Coronavirus (COVID-19)." *Journal of the American Psychiatric Nurses Association* 26, no. 4 (July 2020): 340–343. https://doi.org/10.1177/1078390320919803.

Chronicle of Higher Education Editors. "How to Solve the Student-Disengage- ment Crisis." *Chronicle of Higher Education*, May 11, 2022. https://perma .cc/E98H-B7UN. https://www.chronicle.com/article/how-to-solve-the-stu dent-disengagement-crisis.

Ciciurkaite, Gabriele, Guadalupe Marquez-Velarde, and Robyn Lewis Brown. "Stressors Associated with the COVID-19 Pandemic, Disability, and Mental Health: Considerations from the Intermountain West." *Stress and Health* 38, no. 2 (April 2022): 304–317. https://doi.org/10.1002/smi.3091.

Cleveland Clinic. "Neurodivergent." Accessed April 1, 2023. https://my.cleve landclinic.org/health/symptoms/23154-neurodivergent.

Cohan, Deborah J. "Upholding Rigor at Pandemic U." *Inside Higher Ed*, August 25, 2021. https://perma.cc/NMP8-XZCE. https://www.insidehighered.com /advice/2021/08/25/professors-should-uphold-rigor-when-assessing-stu dents-even-pandemic-opinion.

Cohen, Rachel M. "Are Active Shooter Drills Worth It?" *Vox*, May 28, 2022. https://perma.cc/8NQN-FZVZ. https://www.vox.com/23144105/lockdown -drills-active-shooter-uvalde-robb-texas.

Comtois, Katherine Anne. "A Review of Interventions to Reduce the Prevalence of Parasuicide." *Psychiatric Services* 53, no. 9 (September 2002): 1138–1144. https://doi.org/10.1176/appi.ps.53.9.1138.

Cornell University. "Universal Design for Learning." *Cornell Center for Teaching Innovation.* Accessed March 26, 2023. https://teaching.cornell.edu/teach ing-resources/designing-your-course/universal-design-learning.

Cortland, Matthew. "Why Banning Laptops Is Harmful." *Education in Chemistry,* October 6, 2017. https://perma.cc/9783-J6F3. https://edu.rsc.org/end point/why-banning-laptops-is-harmful/3008076.article.

Costa, Karen Ray. "Is COVID a Collective Trauma?" *Karen Ray Costa,* February 9, 2022. https://perma.cc/2YMH-5Y2Z. https://karenraycosta.medium .com/is-covid-a-collective-trauma-e83bb1c2e2a7.

———. "The Next Phase." *Karen Ray Costa,* May 19, 2021. https://karenraycosta .medium.com/the-next-phase-a7912bc6a453.

———. "Tweet Coining the Term 'Toxic Rigor.'" Twitter, December 9, 2020. Screenshot available upon request.

Cottom, Tressie McMillan. "Everything but the Burden: Publics, Public Scholarship, and Institutions." *Some of Us Are Brave: The Archive,* May 12, 2015. https://perma.cc/2MUQ-DZYY. https://tressiemc.com/uncategorized/every thing-but-the-burden-publics-public-scholarship-and-institutions/.

———. "'Who Do You Think You Are?': When Marginality Meets Academic Microcelebrity." *Ada: A Journal of Gender, New Media, and Technology* 7 (2015). https://doi.org/10.7264/N3319T5T.

Coughlin, Maggie. "10 Things Faculty Need to Understand about Autism." *Inside Higher Ed,* October 20, 2021. https://www.insidehighered.com/ad vice/2021/10/20/lessons-teaching-students-autism-spectrum-opinion.

COVID-19 Mental Disorders Collaborators. "Global Prevalence and Burden of Depressive and Anxiety Disorders in 204 Countries and Territories in 2020 Due to the COVID-19 Pandemic." *The Lancet* 398, no. 10312 (November 2021): 1700–1712. https://doi.org/10.1016/S0140-6736(21)02143-7.

Cowan, Nelson. "Working Memory Underpins Cognitive Development, Learning, and Education." *Educational Psychology Review* 26, no. 2 (June 1, 2014): 197–223. https://doi.org/10.1007/s10648-013-9246-y.

Crocker, Amy F., and Susan N. Smith. "Person-First Language: Are We Practicing What We Preach?" *Journal of Multidisciplinary Healthcare* 12 (February 8, 2019): 125–129. https://doi.org/10.2147/JMDH.S140067.

Curcio, Andrea A., and Mary A. Lynch. "Addressing Social Loafing on Faculty Committees." *Journal of Legal Education* 67, no. 1 (Autumn 2017): 242–262. https://doi.org/10.31228/osf.io/yzgbf.

Czeisler, Mark É., Rashon I. Lane, Emiko Petrosky, Joshua F. Wiley, Aleta Christensen, Rashid Njai, Matthew D. Weaver, et al. "Mental Health, Substance Use, and Suicidal Ideation During the COVID-19 Pandemic—United States, June 24–30, 2020." *Centers for Disease Control Morbidity and*

Mortality Weekly Report 69, no. 32 (August 14, 2020): 1049–1057. https://doi.org/10.15585/mmwr.mm6932a1.

Davey, Graham C. L., and Suzannah Levy. "Catastrophic Worrying: Personal Inadequacy and a Perseverative Iterative Style as Features of the Catastrophizing Process." *Journal of Abnormal Psychology* 107 (1998): 576–586. https://doi.org/10.1037/0021-843X.107.4.576.

Davis, Lennard. "Introduction." In *The Disability Studies Reader*, 2nd ed., edited by Lennard Davis, xv–xvii. New York: Routledge, 2006.

Denial, Catherine J. "A Pedagogy of Kindness." *Hybrid Pedagogy*, August 15, 2019. https://hybridpedagogy.org/pedagogy-of-kindness/.

Deo, Meera E. "Pandemic Pressures on Faculty." *University of Pennsylvania Law Review Online* 170, no. 1 (2022): 127–146.

DeVries, Evan, and The Thompson Policy Institute. "Comparing Mental Illness and Intellectual and Developmental Disabilities." *Chapman University*, August 2, 2016. https://blogs.chapman.edu/tpi/2016/08/02/comparing-mental-illness-and-intellectual-and-developmental-disabilities/.

Dewsbury, Bryan M., Holly J. Swanson, Serena Moseman-Valtierra, and Joshua Caulkins. "Inclusive and Active Pedagogies Reduce Academic Outcome Gaps and Improve Long-Term Performance." *PLOS ONE* 17, no. 6 (June 15, 2022): e0268620. https://doi.org/10.1371/journal.pone.0268620.

Dolmage, Jay Timothy. *Academic Ableism: Disability in Higher Education.* Ann Arbor: University of Michigan Press, 2017.

Dorfman, Doron. "Fear of the Disability Con: Perceptions of Fraud and Special Rights Discourse." *Law and Society Review* 53, no. 4 (December 2019): 1051–1091. https://doi.org/10.1111/lasr.12437.

———. "[Un]Usual Suspects: Deservingness, Scarcity, and Disability Rights." *University of California at Irvine Law Review* 10, no. 2 (2020): 557–618.

Dubey, Pradeep K., and John Geanakoplos. "Grading Exams: 100, 99, 98, . . . Or A, B, C?" *SSRN Scholarly Paper*, Rochester, NY, June 18, 2009. https://doi.org/10.2139/ssrn.1421986.

El-Sabawi, Taleed, and Madison Fields, eds. "The Discounted Labor of BIPOC Students & Faculty." *California Law Review Online* 12, no. 1212849 (2021): 17–29. https://doi.org/10.15779/Z38HX15R7B.

Emerson College Emergency Management. "ALICE Training." *Emerson College.* https://perma.cc/CV28-EEHB. Accessed January 1, 2023. https://emerson.edu/departments/emergency-management/safety-awareness-trainings/alice-training.

Engle, Randall W. "What Is Working Memory Capacity?" In *The Nature of Remembering: Essays in Honor of Robert G. Crowder*, edited by Henry Roediger, James Nairne, Ian Neath, and Aimee Surprenant, 297–314. Washington, DC: American Psychological Association, 2001. https://doi.org/10.1037/10394-016.

Fang, Jenn. "Asian American Student Suicide Rate at MIT Is Quadruple the National Average." *Reappropriate: Asian American Feminism, Politics, and Pop Culture*, May 20, 2015. https://perma.cc/NK6X-V6QU. http://reappropriate.co/2015/05/asian-american-student-suicide-rate-at-mit-is-quadruple-the-national-average/.

Febos, Melissa. "Do You Want to Be Known for Your Writing, or for Your Swift Email Responses?" *Catapult*, March 23, 2017. https://perma.cc/V6ES-B93G. https://catapult.co/stories/do-you-want-to-be-known-for-your-writing-or-for-your-swift-email-responses.

Findijs, Alex. "UNC Chapel Hill Campus Mourns Suicide and Attempted Suicide of Two Students over the Weekend." *World Socialist Web Site*, October 14, 2021. https://perma.cc/R7L4-QJDJ. https://www.wsws.org/en/articles/2021/10/15/unca-015.html.

Flett, Alison L., Mohsen Haghbin, and Timothy A. Pychyl. "Procrastination and Depression from a Cognitive Perspective: An Exploration of the Associations among Procrastinatory Automatic Thoughts, Rumination, and Mindfulness." *Journal of Rational-Emotive & Cognitive-Behavior Therapy* 34, no. 3 (September 2016): 169–186. https://doi.org/10.1007/s10942-016-0235-1.

Ford, Star. "Deep Accessibility." *Ianology*, September 6, 2013. https://perma.cc/AN42-J8TM. https://ianology.wordpress.com/2013/09/06/deep-accessibility/.

Freeman, Scott, Sarah L. Eddy, Miles McDonough, Michelle K. Smith, Nnadozie Okoroafor, Hannah Jordt, and Mary Pat Wenderoth. "Active Learning Increases Student Performance in Science, Engineering, and Mathematics." *Proceedings of the National Academy of Sciences of the United States of America* 111, no. 23 (June 2014): 8410–8415. https://doi.org/10.1073/pnas.1319030111.

Friga, Paul M. "How Much Has Covid Cost Colleges? $183 Billion." *Chronicle of Higher Education*, February 5, 2021. https://perma.cc/6T3B-9596. https://www.chronicle.com/article/how-to-fight-covids-financial-crush.

Fruscione, Joseph, and Kelly J. Baker. "Introduction." In *Succeeding outside the Academy: Career Paths beyond the Humanities, Social Sciences, and STEM*, edited by Joseph Fruscione and Kelly J. Baker, 1–7. Lawrence: University Press of Kansas, 2018.

Gannon, Kevin. "Post-Covid, the Personal Is the Professional." *Chronicle of Higher Education*, April 4, 2022. https://www.chronicle.com/article/postcovid-the-personal-is-the-professional.

———. "Why Calls for a 'Return to Rigor' Are Wrong." *Chronicle of Higher Education*, May 22, 2023. https://www.chronicle.com/article/why-calls-for-a-return-to-rigor-are-wrong.

Garcia, Eric. *We're Not Broken: Changing the Autism Conversation*. Boston: Houghton Mifflin Harcourt, 2021.

Garland-Thomson, Rosemarie. *Extraordinary Bodies: Figuring Physical Disability in American Culture and Literature*. New York: Columbia University Press, 2017.

———. *Staring: How We Look*. New York: Oxford University Press, 2009.

Gordon, Joshua. "One Year In: COVID-19 and Mental Health." *National Institute of Mental Health (NIMH)*, April 9, 2021. https://perma.cc/TYL3-M5F2. https://www.nimh.nih.gov/about/director/messages/2021/one-year-in-covid-19-and-mental-health.

Grant, Adam. "Why We Should Stop Grading Students on a Curve." *New York Times*, September 10, 2016. https://perma.cc/Z6SS-C5DF. https://www.nytimes.com/2016/09/11/opinion/sunday/why-we-should-stop-grading-students-on-a-curve.html.

Grey, Ashe. "Bad Crip: A Probably Not Comprehensive Definition." *Crippled Scholar*, March 14, 2016. https://perma.cc/6N9Q-SU8G. https://crippledscholar.com/2016/03/14/bad-crip-a-probably-not-comprehensive-definition/.

Guarino, Cassandra M., and Victor M. H. Borden. "Faculty Service Loads and Gender: Are Women Taking Care of the Academic Family?" *Research in Higher Education* 58, no. 6 (September 1, 2017): 672–694. https://doi.org/10.1007/s11162-017-9454-2.

Harley, Debra A. "Maids of Academe: African American Women Faculty at Predominately White Institutions." *Journal of African American Studies* 12, no. 1 (March 2008): 19–36. https://doi.org/10.1007/s12111-007-9030-5.

Hayes, Sherrill W., Jennifer L. Priestley, Brian A. Moore, and Herman E. Ray. "Perceived Stress, Work-Related Burnout, and Working from Home before and during COVID-19: An Examination of Workers in the United States." *SAGE Open* 11, no. 4 (October 2021). https://doi.org/10.1177/21582440211058193.

Healthy Minds Network. "Fall 2020 Data Report." *The Healthy Minds Study*, Fall 2020. https://perma.cc/9XWA-2DF8. https://healthymindsnetwork.org/wp-content/uploads/2021/02/HMS-Fall-2020-National-Data-Report.pdf.

Hirschberger, Gilad. "Collective Trauma and the Social Construction of Meaning." *Frontiers in Psychology* 9 (August 10, 2018): 1441. https://doi.org/10.3389/fpsyg.2018.01441.

Hogan, Kelly A., and Viji Sathy. *Inclusive Teaching: Strategies for Promoting Equity in the College Classroom*. Morgantown: West Virginia University Press, 2022.

Hornstein, Gail A. "Why I Dread the Accommodations Talk." *Chronicle of Higher Education*, March 26, 2017. https://perma.cc/PP73-8WKJ. https://www.chronicle.com/article/Why-I-Dread-the-Accommodations/239571.

Howard, Ron, dir. *A Beautiful Mind*. Universal City, CA: Universal Pictures, 2001.

Hubbard, Nicholas A., Joanna L. Hutchison, Monroe Turner, Janelle Montroy, Ryan P. Bowles, and Bart Rypma. "Depressive Thoughts Limit Working Memory Capacity in Dysphoria." *Cognition and Emotion* 30, no. 2 (February 17, 2016): 193–209. https://doi.org/10.1080/02699931.2014.991694.

Hull, Laura, K. V. Petrides, Carrie Allison, Paula Smith, Simon Baron-Cohen, Meng-Chuan Lai, and William Mandy. "'Putting on My Best Normal': Social Camouflaging in Adults with Autism Spectrum Conditions." *Journal of Autism and Developmental Disorders* 47, no. 8 (August 2017): 2519–2534. https://doi.org/10.1007/s10803-017-3166-5.

Hupfeld, Kathleen E., Tessa R. Abagis, and Priti Shah. "Living 'in the Zone': Hyperfocus in Adult ADHD." *ADHD Attention Deficit and Hyperactivity Disorders* 11, no. 2 (June 1, 2019): 191–208. https://doi.org/10.1007/s12402-018-0272-y.

Imad, Mays. "Hope Matters." *Inside Higher Ed*, March 17, 2020. https://perma.cc/FH89-LYED. https://www.insidehighered.com/advice/2020/03/17/10-strategies-support-students-and-help-them-learn-during-coronavirus-crisis.

Jack, Jordynn, and Viji Sathy. "It's Time to Cancel the Word 'Rigor.'" *Chronicle of Higher Education*, September 24, 2021. https://perma.cc/ERV2-5DAW. https://www.chronicle.com/article/its-time-to-cancel-the-word-rigor.

Janicki, Matthew P., James A. Hendrix, and Philip McCallion. "Examining Older Adults with Neuroatypical Conditions for MCI/Dementia: Barriers and Recommendations of the Neuroatypical Conditions Expert Consultative Panel." *Alzheimer's & Dementia: Diagnosis, Assessment & Disease Monitoring* 14, no. 1 (July 8, 2022): e12335. https://doi.org/10.1002/dad2.12335.

Janowski, Elizabeth Pham. "Sent Away." *Chronicle of Higher Education*, June 27, 2022. https://www.chronicle.com/article/sent-away.

Katherine, Anne. "Create Boundaries." *Your Cherished Life*. https://perma.cc/A6PW-LK2B. Accessed October 6, 2022. https://1annekatherine.com/httpwp-mep39g1w-z/.

——. *Where to Draw the Line: How to Set Healthy Boundaries Every Day*. New York: Touchstone, 2012.

Kaul, Kate. "Risking Experience: Disability, Precarity, and Disclosure." In *Negotiating Disability: Disclosure and Higher Education*, edited by Stephanie L. Kerschbaum, Laura T. Eisenman, and James M. Jones, 171–187. Ann Arbor: University of Michigan Press, 2017. https://doi.org/10.3998/mpub.9426902.

Kelly, Owen. "What Are Anxiety Disorders?" *Verywell Mind*, May 14, 2022. https://perma.cc/RXB2-ZVZC. https://www.verywellmind.com/anxiety-disorder-2510539.

Kercood, Suneeta, Janice A. Grskovic, Devender Banda, and Jasmine Begeske. "Working Memory and Autism: A Review of Literature." *Research in Autism Spectrum Disorders* 8, no. 10 (October 1, 2014): 1316–1332. https://doi.org/10.1016/j.rasd.2014.06.011.

Kesslen, Ben. "UNC Chapel Hill Cancels Classes Tuesday amid Two Suicide Investigations." *NBC News*, October 11, 2021. https://perma.cc/WH38-Z434. https://www.nbcnews.com/news/us-news/unc-chapel-hill-cancels-classes-tuesday-amid-two-suicide-investigations-n1281229.

Kim, Joseph A., Peter Szatmari, Susan E. Bryson, David L. Streiner, and Freda J. Wilson. "The Prevalence of Anxiety and Mood Problems among Children with Autism and Asperger Syndrome." *Autism* 4, no. 2 (June 1, 2000): 117–132. https://doi.org/10.1177/1362361300004002002.

Kuehn, Bridget M. "Clinician Shortage Exacerbates Pandemic-Fueled 'Mental Health Crisis.'" *JAMA* 327, no. 22 (June 14, 2022): 2179–2181. https://doi.org/10.1001/jama.2022.8661.

Lashuel, Hilal A. "Mental Health in Academia: What about Faculty?" *ELife* 9 (January 8, 2020): e54551. https://doi.org/10.7554/eLife.54551.

Link, Bruce G., and Jo C. Phelan. "Conceptualizing Stigma." *Annual Review of Sociology* 27, no. 1 (August 2001): 363–385. https://doi.org/10.1146/annurev.soc.27.1.363.

Link, Bruce G., Jo C. Phelan, Michaeline Bresnahan, Ann Stueve, and Bernice A. Pescosolido. "Public Conceptions of Mental Illness: Labels, Causes, Dangerousness, and Social Distance." *American Journal of Public Health* 89, no. 9 (September 1999): 1328–1333. https://doi.org/10.2105/AJPH.89.9.1328.

Litman, Robert E. "Medical-Legal Aspects of Suicide." *Washburn Law Journal* 6, no. 2 (Winter 1967): 395–401.

López, Rachel. "Unentitled: The Power of Designation in the Legal Academy." *Rutgers University Law Review* 73, no. 3 (Spring 2021): 923–932.

Low, Keith. "What Is Executive Function?" *Verywell Mind*, September 27, 2020. https://www.verywellmind.com/what-are-executive-functions-20463.

Lu, Thomas, and Sylvie Douglis. "Don't Be Scared to Talk about Disabilities: Here's What to Know and What to Say." *NPR*, February 22, 2022. https://perma.cc/D5KU-A8C3. https://www.npr.org/2022/02/18/1081713756/disability-disabled-people-offensive-better-word.

Macfarlane, Katherine. "Accommodation Discrimination (Preprint)." *American University Law Review* 72 (2023). https://doi.org/10.2139/ssrn.4190587.

———. "Disability without Documentation." *Fordham Law Review* 90, no. 1 (2021): 59–102.

Mak, Arthur D. P., Sue Lee, Nancy A. Sampson, Yesica Albor, Jordi Alonso, Randy P. Auerbach, Harald Baumeister, et al. "ADHD Comorbidity Structure and Impairment: Results of the WHO World Mental Health Surveys International College Student Project (WMH-ICS)." *Journal of Attention Disorders* 26, no. 8 (June 1, 2022): 1078–1096. https://doi.org/10.1177/10870547211057275.

Malesic, Jonathan. "My College Students Are Not OK." *New York Times*, May 13, 2022. https://perma.cc/V65W-PXXS. https://www.nytimes.com/2022/05/13/opinion/college-university-remote-pandemic.html.

Maslach, Christina, Wilmar B. Schaufeli, and Michael P. Leiter. "Job Burnout." *Annual Review of Psychology* 52, no. 1 (February 2001): 397–422. https://doi.org/10.1146/annurev.psych.52.1.397.

McClure, Kevin R. "Don't Blame the Pandemic for Worker Discontent." *Chronicle of Higher Education*, May 27, 2022. https://www.chronicle.com/article/dont-blame-the-pandemic-for-worker-discontent.

McClure, Kevin R., and Alisa Hicklin Fryar. "The Great Faculty Disengagement." *Chronicle of Higher Education*, January 19, 2022. https://perma.cc/QXP5-GKJH. https://www.chronicle.com/article/the-great-faculty-disengagement.

McCrossin, Robert. "Finding the True Number of Females with Autistic Spectrum Disorder by Estimating the Biases in Initial Recognition and Clinical Diagnosis." *Children (Basel, Switzerland)* 9, no. 2 (February 17, 2022): 272. https://doi.org/10.3390/children9020272.

McDermott, Victoria, Teresa Heinz Housel, Leandra Hernández, Erica Knotts, Amy May, and Stevie M. Munz, eds. *On the Front Lines: Women Educators' Experiences during the COVID-19 Pandemic.* Lanham, MD: Lexington Books, 2023.

McGuire, Joan M., and Sally S. Scott. "An Approach for Inclusive College Teaching: Universal Design for Instruction." *Learning Disabilities: A Multidisciplinary Journal* 14, no. 1 (2006): 21–32.

Meek, Andy. "NRA's Wayne LaPierre: 'Good Guys with Guns' Could Have Stopped Navy Yard Shooting." *Time*, September 22, 2013. http://nation.time.com/2013/09/22/nras-wayne-lapierre-good-guys-with-guns-could-have-stopped-navy-yard-shooting/.

Meeks, Kasey, Amy Sutton Peak, and Adam Dreihaus. "Depression, Anxiety, and Stress among Students, Faculty, and Staff." *Journal of American College Health* 71, no. 2 (February 12, 2023): 348–354. https://doi.org/10.1080/07448481.2021.1891913.

Miller, Julius. "Stanford Responds to Suicide Crisis After 4th Student in 13 Months Takes Her Own Life." *Los Angeles Magazine*, March 11, 2022. https://perma.cc/83A7-CZ5E. https://www.lamag.com/article/stanford-responds-to-suicide-crisis-after-4th-student-in-13-months-takes-her-own-life/.

Mueller, Pam A., and Daniel M. Oppenheimer. "The Pen Is Mightier than the Keyboard: Advantages of Longhand over Laptop Note Taking." *Psychological Science* 25, no. 6 (June 1, 2014): 1159–1168. https://doi.org/10.1177/0956797614524581.

Muscatelli, Anton. "Universities Must Overhaul the Toxic Working Culture for Academic Researchers." *The Guardian*, January 15, 2020. https://perma.cc/MM58-Y87N.https://www.theguardian.com/education/2020/jan/15/universities-must-overhaul-the-toxic-working-culture-for-academic-researchers.

Napp, Abigail, and Harsha Nahata. "When Colleges Fail on Mental Health."

NYCITY NewsService of the CUNY Craig Newmark Graduate School of Journalism, May 5, 2020. https://perma.cc/N45N-MBTA. https://campusmentalhealth.nycitynewsservice.com/.

National Center for Education Statistics. "A Majority of College Students with Disabilities Do Not Inform School, New NCES Data Show." *National Center for Education Statistics*, April 26, 2022. https://nces.ed.gov/whatsnew/press_releases/4_26_2022.asp.

National Institute of Mental Health. "Any Anxiety Disorder." Accessed March 23, 2023. https://www.nimh.nih.gov/health/statistics/any-anxiety-disorder.

Neff, Kristin D. "Self-Compassion: An Alternative Conceptualization of a Healthy Attitude Toward Oneself." *Self and Identity* 2, no. 2 (April 2003): 85–101. https://doi.org/10.1080/15298860309032.

Neff, Kristin D., Ya-Ping Hsieh, and Kullaya Dejitterat. "Self-Compassion, Achievement Goals, and Coping with Academic Failure." *Self and Identity* 4, no. 3 (July 2005): 263–287. https://doi.org/10.1080/13576500444000317.

Nolen-Hoeksema, Susan, Blair E. Wisco, and Sonja Lyubomirsky. "Rethinking Rumination." *Perspectives on Psychological Science* 3, no. 5 (September 2008): 400–424. https://doi.org/10.1111/j.1745-6924.2008.00088.x.

Olsen-Reeder, Vini. "Commentary: 'Plumbing Leaks: The Post-Pandemic Neoliberal Turn of Tertiary Students.'" *New Zealand Journal of Educational Studies*, December 15, 2022. https://doi.org/10.1007/s40841-022-00272-1.

O'Toole, Corbett. "Disclosing Our Relationships to Disabilities: An Invitation for Disability Studies Scholars." *Disability Studies Quarterly* 33, no. 2 (March 27, 2013). https://doi.org/10.18061/dsq.v33i2.3708.

Padilla, Amado M. "Ethnic Minority Scholars, Research, and Mentoring: Current and Future Issues." *Educational Researcher* 23, no. 4 (May 1994): 24–27. https://doi.org/10.3102/0013189X023004024.

Perini, Giulia, Matteo Cotta Ramusino, Elena Sinforiani, Sara Bernini, Roberto Petrachi, and Alfredo Costa. "Cognitive Impairment in Depression: Recent Advances and Novel Treatments." *Neuropsychiatric Disease and Treatment* 15 (May 2019): 1249–1258. https://doi.org/10.2147/NDT.S199746.

Phelps, Fiona G., Gwyneth Doherty-Sneddon, and Hannah Warnock. "Helping Children Think: Gaze Aversion and Teaching." *British Journal of Developmental Psychology* 24, no. 3 (2006): 577–588. https://doi.org/10.1348/026151005X49872.

Pinder-Amaker, Stephanie. "Identifying the Unmet Needs of College Students on the Autism Spectrum." *Harvard Review of Psychiatry* 22, no. 2 (2014): 125–137. https://doi.org/10.1097/HRP.0000000000000032.

Pope-Ruark, Rebecca. *Unraveling Faculty Burnout: Pathways to Reckoning and Renewal*. Baltimore: Johns Hopkins University Press, 2022. https://doi.org/10.56021/9781421445137.

Poplett, Emilie. "Carolina Launches 24/7 Hotline to Support Student Mental

Health." *The University of North Carolina at Chapel Hill*, August 19, 2019. https://perma.cc/AX54-KQ7V. https://www.unc.edu/posts/2019/08/19/carolina-launches-24-7-hotline-to-support-student-mental-health/.

Potter, Claire Bond. "The Hard Truths of the Academic-Labor Crisis." *Chronicle of Higher Education*, November 17, 2022. https://www.chronicle.com/article/the-hard-truths-of-the-academic-labor-crisis.

Prendergast, Catherine. "On the Rhetorics of Mental Disability." In *Embodied Rhetorics: Disability in Language and Culture*, edited by James C. Wilson and Cynthia Lewiecki-Wilson, 45–60. Carbondale: Southern Illinois University Press, 2003.

Price, Devon. "Laziness Does Not Exist." *Human Parts*, March 23, 2018. https://perma.cc/LZ8J-LXWU.https://humanparts.medium.com/laziness-does-not-exist-3af27e312d01.

———. *Laziness Does Not Exist: A Defense of the Exhausted, Exploited, and Overworked*. New York: Simon and Schuster, 2021.

Price, Margaret. *Mad at School: Rhetorics of Mental Disability and Academic Life*. Ann Arbor: University of Michigan Press, 2011.

Price, Margaret, Mark S. Salzer, Amber O'Shea, and Stephanie L. Kerschbaum. "Disclosure of Mental Disability by College and University Faculty: The Negotiation of Accommodations, Supports, and Barriers." *Disability Studies Quarterly* 37, no. 2 (June 1, 2017). https://doi.org/10.18061/dsq.v37i2.5487.

Pryal, Katie Rose Guest. "Disclosure Blues: Should You Tell Colleagues about Your Mental Illness?" *Chronicle of Higher Education*, June 13, 2014. http://dx.doi.org/10.2139/ssrn.4158926.

———. "Do One Thing." *Women in Higher Education* 28, no. 2 (2019): 13. https://doi.org/10.1002/whe.20673.

———. "Front-Line Faculty and Systemic Burnout: Why More Faculty Should Attend to Law Students' Mental Health and the Inequities Caused by Faculty Who Opt Out." *Legal Writing: The Journal of the Legal Writing Institute* 27, no. 1 (2023): 199–221.

———. "Heller's Scapegoats." *North Carolina Law Review* 93, no. 5 (June 2015): 1439–1474.

———. "How the TSA Perpetuates Harmful Mental Health Stigmas." *The Establishment*, May 12, 2016. https://perma.cc/7E2J-78SC. https://medium.com/the-establishment/how-the-tsa-perpetuates-harmful-mental-health-stigmas-90f531962158.

———. How to Write Publicly about Rape." In *Even If You're Broken: Essays on Sexual Assault and #MeToo*, by Katie Rose Guest Pryal. Chapel Hill, NC: Blue Crow Books, 2019.

———. *Life of the Mind Interrupted: Essays on Mental Health and Disability in Higher Education*. Chapel Hill, NC: Blue Crow Books, 2017.

———. "My Disability Story Isn't for Your Catharsis." *The Establishment*,

September 25, 2018. https://perma.cc/V7Z8-6UGR. https://theestablish
ment.co/my-disability-story-isnt-for-your-catharsis/index.html.

———. "The World Doesn't Bend for Disabled Kids (or Disabled Parents)." *Catapult*, July 10, 2018. https://perma.cc/ZX2L-JX9E. https://catapult.co/sto
ries/the-world-doesnt-bend-for-disabled-kids-or-disabled-parents.

Pryal, Katie Rose Guest, and Jordynn Jack. "When You Talk about Banning
Laptops, You Throw Disabled Students under the Bus." *Huffington Post*, November 27, 2017. http://dx.doi.org/10.2139/ssrn.4166867.

Randall, David. "Don't Cancel Rigor." *National Association of Scholars*, November 4, 2021. https://perma.cc/7DL2-Z42Q. https://www.nas.org/blogs/arti
cle/dont-cancel-rigor.

Reevy, Gretchen M., and Grace Deason. "Predictors of Depression, Stress, and
Anxiety among Non-Tenure Track Faculty." *Frontiers in Psychology* 5, no. 701
(July 8, 2014): 1–17. https://doi.org/10.3389/fpsyg.2014.00701.

Richards, Lamar. "Lamar Richards, Tweet as UNC Student Body President,
Stating Students Need a Break from Classes the Day after the Announce-
ment of Multiple Student Deaths by Suicide." Twitter, October 10, 2021.
Screenshot available upon request.

Romano, Aja. "A History of 'Wokeness.'" *Vox*, October 9, 2020. https://perma
.cc/33TM-4SEH. https://www.vox.com/culture/21437879/stay-woke-woke
ness-history-origin-evolution-controversy.

Russo, Anthony and Joe, dir. *Captain America: Civil War*. Burbank, CA: Marvel
Studios, 2016.

Samli, Ayla, and Katie Rose Guest Pryal. "Accommodations Are Not Accessibility:
An Interview with Katie Rose Guest Pryal." *The Rumpus*, September 21, 2022.
https://perma.cc/JR6G-5VTM. https://therumpus.net/2022/09/21/accom
modations-are-not-accessibility-an-interview-with-katie-rose-guest-pryal/.

Sarrett, Jennifer C. "Autism and Accommodations in Higher Education: Insights from the Autism Community." *Journal of Autism and Developmental
Disorders* 48, no. 3 (March 2018): 679–693. https://doi.org/10.1007/s10803
-017-3353-4.

Schendel, Sarah J. "Due Dates in the Real World: Extensions, Equity, and the
Hidden Curriculum." *Georgetown Journal of Legal Ethics* 35, no. 2 (2022):
203–233.

———. "The Pandemic Syllabus." *Denver Law Review Forum*, November 30,
2020. https://perma.cc/2FUH-DNUJ. https://www.denverlawreview.org/dlr
-online-article/pandemicsyllabus.

Schumann, Abel. "Persistence of Population Shocks: Evidence from the Occupation of West Germany after World War II." *American Economic Journal:
Applied Economics* 6, no. 3 (July 2014): 189–205.

Singer, Judy. "'Why Can't You Be Normal for Once in Your Life?': From a 'Problem with No Name' to the Emergence of a New Category of Difference." In

Disability Discourse, edited by Mairian Corker and Sally French, 59–67. Philadelphia: Open University Press, 1999.

Solomon, Andrew. *The Noonday Demon: An Atlas of Depression*. New York: Scribner, 2001.

Stimpunks. "Eye Contact and Neurodiversity." *Stimpunks Foundation*, March 2, 2023. https://stimpunks.org/eye-contact/.

Styron, William. *Darkness Visible: A Memoir of Madness*. New York: Random House, 1990.

Supiano, Beckie. "A Different Way of Thinking about Rigor." *Chronicle of Higher Education*, November 18, 2021. https://www.chronicle.com/newsletter/teaching/2021-11-18.

———. "The Redefinition of Rigor." *Chronicle of Higher Education*, March 29, 2022. https://perma.cc/2XGW-WTJS. https://www.chronicle.com/article/the-redefinition-of-rigor.

———. "Worried about Cutting Content? This Study Suggests It's OK." *Chronicle of Higher Education*, July 7, 2022. https://www.chronicle.com/newsletter/teaching/2022-07-07.

Tal Young, Ilanit, Alana Iglewicz, Danielle Glorioso, Nicole Lanouette, Kathryn Seay, Manjusha Ilapakurti, and Sidney Zisook. "Suicide Bereavement and Complicated Grief." *Dialogues in Clinical Neuroscience* 14, no. 2 (June 30, 2012): 177–186. https://doi.org/10.31887/DCNS.2012.14.2/iyoung.

Thorp, H. Holden. "Inclusion Doesn't Lower Standards." *Science* 377, no. 6602 (July 8, 2022): 129. https://doi.org/10.1126/science.add7259.

Toutain, Christopher. "Barriers to Accommodations for Students with Disabilities in Higher Education: A Literature Review." *Journal of Postsecondary Education and Disability* 32, no. 3 (Fall 2019): 297–310.

Urry, Heather L., Chelsea S. Crittle, Victoria A. Floerke, Michael Z. Leonard, Clinton S. Perry, Naz Akdilek, Erica R. Albert, et al. "Don't Ditch the Laptop Just Yet: A Direct Replication of Mueller and Oppenheimer's (2014) Study 1 Plus Mini Meta-Analyses across Similar Studies." *Psychological Science* 32, no. 3 (March 1, 2021): 326–339. https://doi.org/10.1177/0956797620965541.

Wang, Esmé Weijun. *The Collected Schizophrenias: Essays*. Minneapolis, MN: Graywolf Press, 2019.

Westervelt, Eric. "Mental Health and Police Violence: How Crisis Intervention Teams Are Failing." *NPR*, September 18, 2020. https://perma.cc/U7CM-8ZU2. https://www.npr.org/2020/09/18/913229469/mental-health-and-police-violence-how-crisis-intervention-teams-are-failing.

White, Susan W., Thomas H. Ollendick, and Bethany C. Bray. "College Students on the Autism Spectrum: Prevalence and Associated Problems." *Autism* 15, no. 6 (November 1, 2011): 683–701. https://doi.org/10.1177/1362361310393363.

Wisdom, Maria LaMonaca. "What Is the Real Cost of Academe's Fixation on Productivity?" *Chronicle of Higher Education*, May 5, 2022. https://www

.chronicle.com/article/what-is-the-real-cost-of-academes-fixation-on-pro ductivity.

Wong, Alice. *Year of the Tiger: An Activist's Life*. New York: Vintage, 2022.

World Health Organization News. "Burn-Out an 'Occupational Phenomenon': International Classification of Diseases." *World Health Organization*, May 28, 2019. https://www.who.int/news/item/28-05-2019-burn-out-an-occu pational-phenomenon-international-classification-of-diseases.

Yergeau, M. Remi. "Clinically Significant Disturbance: On Theorists Who The orize Theory of Mind." *Disability Studies Quarterly* 33, no. 4 (September 5, 2013). https://doi.org/10.18061/dsq.v33i4.3876.

Young, Stella. "I'm Not Your Inspiration, Thank You Very Much." *TEDxSydney*, June 9, 2014. https://perma.cc/W6P3-ZZVX. https://www.ted.com/talks /stella_young_i_m_not_your_inspiration_thank_you_very_much.

Index

failure and, 50
   toxic, 48–49, 50, 52
failure, 25, 154
   fear of, 50, 155
   higher education and, 49
   overwork and, 50
   perfectionism and, 50
   reframing, 49–50
   rigor and, 105
Fang, Jenn, 96
fatigue, 8, 40, 153
Febos, Melissa, 60
feedback, 49, 79, 119, 149, 173
   collective, 164
   individual, 164
   peer, 130–131
front-line faculty, 98, 146–148, 168
   burdens for, 141
   care from, 139
   help from, 147
   marginalized groups and, 140
   mental health communities and, 142
   people of color as, 21
   retaining, 148
   student communities and, 146
   support from, 21, 147
Fryar, Alisa Hicklin: disengagement and, 43–44

Gannon, Kevin, 109, 111, 159
Garcia, Eric, 128, 137, 165
Garland-Thomson, Rosemarie, 9
gaze aversion, 133. *See also under* autism spectrum disorder; neurodivergent
gender, 80
   faculty positions and, 57
   work and, 141
generalized anxiety disorder (GAD), 3, 22
Georgetown University, 111
good-hard work, 109, 110
Gordon, Joshua A., 30
grading, 26, 136, 164
   absolute, 116
   anxiety and, 24
   on curve, 116
   toxic, 116
Graduate and Professional Student Government, 101

Grandview University, Teaching Center, 109
Grey, Ashe: on bad crip, 8–9
guilt, 25, 49, 55
   shame and, 155

Harley, Debra A., 57
Harris, DeShun, 57
headaches, 68, 69
health issues, 29
   overwork and, 50
Healthy Minds Fall 2020 Data Report (HMS), 99
Healthy Minds Study, 95
higher education employment, 69, 78, 80, 140
   insecure, xiii, 20, 70
Hirschberger, Gilad, 31
Historically Black Colleges and Universities (HBCUs), 57
Hogan, Kelly A., 131, 132
Hornstein, Gail A., 119, 120, 121
Housel, Teresa Heinz, 147, 164

ICD-11. *See* International Classification of Diseases, 11th edition
identity, xiii, 2, 134, 142, 158
   disabled, 8, 11, 34, 45, 96
   normate, 34
   subordinate, 68
   suicide and, 96
Imad, Mays, 110
inclusion, 16, 35, 157, 158
   defining, xiii
   language of, 2
   teaching, 157, 159
Inclusive Teaching: Strategies for Promoting Equity in the College Classroom (Hogan and Sathy), 131
injustice
   epistemic, 67–69
   social, 106
   systemic, 107
Inside Higher Ed, 97, 106
institutional solutions, 44, 153
intellectual and developmental disabilities (IDDs), 5
intellectual growth, 110, 112
intellectual property, abuse of, 168